FRCA Survival Guide

D1341237

To Gill, Emma and Abigail

FRCA Survival Guide

S. M. Yentis BSc MBBS MD FRCA
Consultant Anaesthetist and Director of
Obstetric Anaesthesia,
Chelsea and Westminster Hospital,
London, UK

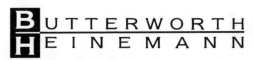

BUTTERWORTH
HEINEMANN

OXFORD   BOSTON   JOHANNESBURG   MELBOURNE   NEW DELHI   SINGAPORE

Butterworth-Heinemann
Linacre House, Jordan Hill, Oxford OX2 8DP
225 Wildwood Avenue, Woburn, MA 01801-2041
A division of Reed Educational and Professional Publishing Ltd

℞ A member of the Reed Elsevier plc group

First published 1998

British Library Cataloguing in Publication Data

A catalogue record for this book is available from the British Library

ISBN 0 7506 3718 8

Typeset in 11/12pt Times by Keyword Typesetting Services Ltd
Printed and bound in Great Britain by Biddles Ltd, Guildford and King's Lynn

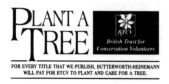

Contents

Preface

Like it or not, examinations are a standard and widely used method of assessing knowledge and competence to practise in medicine. Countless papers, monographs and books have been written about the theory of education applied to the practice of medicine, and the validity or otherwise of exams and other methods of assessment. However, the average trainee anaesthetist has little time or interest in such weighty matters, and has instead to deal with the reality of facing and getting through the FRCA examination within a certain period of training. This two-part hurdle has become central to the 'seamless' training that has dominated recent changes in postgraduate medical education; it lurks in the shadows throughout the trainee years and has the ability to disrupt even the most structured and ordered lifestyle. It also has the distinct property of swooping down on its unsuspecting victims, finding them totally unprepared and often panic-stricken.*

There are many books aimed at exam candidates offering advice and examples directed at specific parts of the FRCA exam, e.g. multiple choice questions, vivas, etc. These are primarily concerned with the content of the exam (how to tackle the subjects examined in) rather than with exam technique itself. However, organising your time, planning revision and developing exam technique are possibly more important than in-depth knowledge of the subject itself, and yet there is little advice available on how to do this. This book is aimed at all anaesthetists contemplating the Primary or Final FRCA and attempts to offer advice on the nature of the beast and how to tackle it. It is intended to be read as a prelude to getting down to proper exam preparation, partly as a relatively undemanding way of easing the guilt that perhaps you should be doing something 'exammy' by now, but also to help plan for the forthcoming months. It is a distillation of the

---

* The sound of distant elephants: you only realise the rumbling has become much louder when you are about to be trampled on.

good advice that I have received as an exam candidate over the years (and now give to new candidates), and advice received or given by various colleagues which has seemed particularly useful. The suggestions have generally been well received by exam candidates in the past and indeed their comments have been the main impetus for this project.

This book does not represent the definitive method of preparing for the FRCA since there is no definitive method, and I have no doubt that there will be many who disagree with its content. Indeed, I am certain that a major criticism from those wiser and older than myself will be that this book is an attempt to offer candidates a short-cut around the requirement for hard graft, blood, sweat and tears, and that we should be training highly-skilled and knowledgeable anaesthetists, not tricksters who can bluff their way through the exams. However, I have seen highly-skilled and knowledgeable anaesthetists fail to get through the exams because they can't negotiate their way through the exam process, and I have seen hopeless clinical anaesthetists get by because they can. I do not question the need for a good grounding in basic science and other important aspects of knowledge on which clinical anaesthesia relies, just the way in which otherwise capable candidates consistently shoot themselves in the foot when the big day arrives.

So why listen to me? I've never been an FRCA examiner (and possibly my chances of being one have taken something of a dive with this publication) but I have sat the FRCA once or twice and have been involved in one way or another in both informal and formal education as a trainer, both within and outside medicine, since my early teens. To be honest, I can think of no really compelling reason, except that the content of this book has served me well over the years, and I hope a few others too. It will not make you a better person, help you lose weight or make you rich, but I hope it will help a little, if only to get you in the right frame of mind for the oncoming onslaught. The style is deliberately non-scientific and, I hope, not too patronising. Please write and tell me if I have got it wrong.

S. M. Yentis

Acknowledgements

I owe sincere thanks to those teachers and helpers who have guided me up to, and occasionally through, various exams over the years. I am also grateful to various trainee and consultant colleagues for the helpful advice, comments on early drafts and exam stories, and to Mrs Maureen Fortier for typing the manuscript. I also thank Dr A. Wolff for describing to me his method of answering multiple choice questions, which I have developed as described in Chapter 3 with his permission. Finally, I wish to thank the President and Board of Examiners at the Royal College of Anaesthetists for the efforts they have made, and are making, to ensure that the FRCA exam is everything it ought to be, i.e. fair, open and honest. Having observed both parts of the FRCA exam, I have been converted from a bitter and twisted cynic to a great supporter of their achievements.

1

Introduction

Candidates have one thing in common: the last thing they need on top of the pressures of work, being on-call, financial or social problems and general worries about the future, is an exam. Until recently, anaesthetists had an extra level of stress compared to their non-anaesthetic colleagues: having to cope with a three part exam instead of two parts for the other specialties. The only good aspect of this from the anaesthetists' point of view was that it reinforced the smug superiority and arrogance that most anaesthetists have anyway. Since the FRCA exam has been reorganised, its syllabus clearly defined and its two parts linked more closely with the structured training, candidates ought to feel more reassured than previously. However, there is now the added pressure of a more clearly defined and limited time period during which they must achieve success and the knowledge that they may be stuck or held back from a planned rotation if they fail. Either way, the furrowed brow and nervous twitch of the anaesthetist who has yet to pass the FRCA exam are well known physical signs to more experienced colleagues.

There exists amongst exam candidates the myth of the Ideal Student, based partly on fact and partly on the mystique attached to successful candidates who apparently do no work at all. These people float around seemingly untouched by the normal worries that afflict the rest, claim to read only the odd article every now and then and yet sail through every test and exam with the best marks ever recorded. There are two explanations for this behaviour: the person is either a very good liar and actor or truly brilliant. Whichever it is, everybody else has the right to hate them bitterly. In fact, the former explanation is more likely to be true, even if put rather

unkindly, since even the brightest of people still need to prepare and study before an exam, especially one with as wide a
scope as most postgraduate exams. Whilst some people are
better than others at doing this, the general processes one has
to go through are essentially the same.

There are many ways in which prospective candidates can
improve their chances of passing the exam: general support;
improving exam technique; and acquiring and improving
practical skills and knowledge. General support is often overlooked but is extremely important. It includes preparing
everybody around you for the fact that you are going to be
under great strain in the near future and will become impos-
sible to live with or to know. It also includes teaming up with
fellow trainees and pooling resources wherever possible. You
will need to rely on each other for exam practice, swapping of
tips and hints, etc. You also need to talk about the exam to
your more senior colleagues so that the whole department is
right behind you. Improving your exam technique involves
planning your revision and knowing and practising the various parts of the exams, as discussed later. Knowing what to
expect and when to expect it can make a huge difference to
your performance on the day. Lastly the acquisition of skills
and knowledge means the subject itself must be covered and
fitted into the exam framework – you need to get used to
thinking in an exam orientated way from quite early on, so
that each encounter with patients or colleagues can be ruth-
lessly exploited to extract every last scrap of learning potential from it.

Examiners

Contrary to popular belief, examiners are normal people who
do what they do for a number of reasons. Kudos, boredom or
simply as a means of getting out of the operating theatre have
all been suggested, but most if not all examiners do it because
they feel that it is important to maintain standards of practice
of anaesthesia; that the FRCA exam is the best way we have
of doing that at present; and that it is their duty to become

involved. Being an examiner is generally hard work and requires great commitment, and attracts little in the way of thanks from those actually taking the exams (in a similar vein, when did you last see a motorist thanking a traffic warden?). The selection of examiners is via journal announcements; various factors affect their acceptance including the individual's particular skills and location. The final say in who should be accepted rests with the College Council, based on the recommendations of the Examinations Committee. Traditionally, examiners have 'graduated' from the earlier parts of the exam to the later ones, but this is no longer the case; examiners may now apply for vacancies on either the Primary or Final. Examiners are offered the opportunity to relinquish their position or change parts of the exam each year. The term of office is now 8 years although it used to be 12 years; occasionally examiners may be invited back to fill in for emergencies such as acute shortages. Not all examiners are involved in each sitting of the exam.

Although many examiners are academic anaesthetists, there is not a minimum quota and you could find yourself face to face with a Professor of Anaesthetics from a teaching centre or a Consultant from a district general hospital. These days examiners are offered a great deal of guidance and support for the exam and there is ongoing assessment and audit of examiners' performance, so increasingly examiners are coming under similar stresses and pressures to those of the candidates themselves. There is no doubt that some examiners are more 'hawkish' whilst others are more 'dovish', but that is true of life anyway and the pairing of hawks with doves and the move towards standardising the exam should minimise any effect this has on an individual candidate's results.

So, just like candidates, the last thing examiners need on top of the pressures of work, being on-call, financial or social problems and general worries about the future, is an exam. The task of the candidate, therefore, is to make life as easy as possible for these poor kindly folk and in so doing, ease their own passage towards examinerdom.

The FRCA exam

The first specialist anaesthetic exam was the Diploma in Anaesthetics (DA), first awarded in 1935 and intended for anaesthetists who had been practising for at least 2 years and who had administered at least 2000 anaesthetics (obviously incompatible with today's post-Calman requirements). This was later changed to 1 year's residence in an approved hospital. In 1947, a two-part exam was introduced to bring it into line with other specialties and to promote the standing of anaesthesia in the new NHS. In 1953, this exam became the Fellowship of the Faculty of Anaesthetists, which at the time was based at the Royal College of Surgeons of England (hence the FFARCS examination, affectionally known as the Free For All Receptions, Cocktails and Socials). In 1984, the DA became the first part of the new three-part FFARCS exam, having been a separate qualification until then. In 1989, the FFARCS became the FCAnaes exam (Fellowship of the College of Anaesthetists) following the establishment of a separate College of Anaesthetists. This College was granted Royal status in 1992 and thus the exam became known by its current name, the FRCA (Fellowship of the Royal College of Anaesthetists).

All this goes to illustrate the fact that the FRCA exam has had a checkered history, and what it is and what it stands for has caused almost as much confusion to its candidates as has the subject matter of the exam. The original DA was seen as something of an apprenticeship; the original two-part FFARCS was viewed with extreme fear and loathing by most people who took it (especially the formidable old Primary, for which, according to many eye witnesses, the connection between basic science and anaesthesia could be raised to new heights of irrelevance). The three-part exam saw many changes and improvements in its structure and administration, and served as a suitable stepping stone for the new and improved two-part exam which began in 1996/ 1997. At the moment, about 750–800 candidates sit each part of the exam per year. The written papers of both parts may be sat provincially as well as in London, depending on demand;

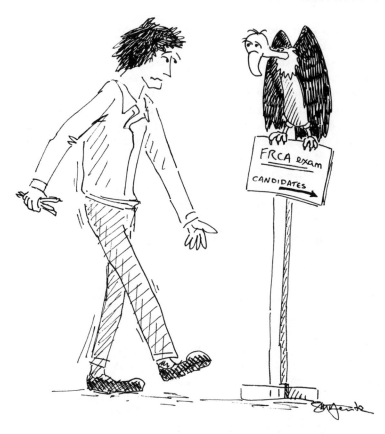

sites include Manchester, Scotland (Glasgow or Edinburgh), the South-West (Bristol or Cardiff) and occasionally Belfast.

Regulations

Detailed regulations for the FRCA are published by the College and any prospective candidate must obtain these and study them well. In brief, candidates may sit the Primary if they have full or provisional GMC registration, have registered with the College as a postgraduate anaesthetic trainee and have completed at least 1 year's satisfactory anaesthetic training as an SHO in a College-approved hospital (College Tutors will advise that 18 months is preferred).

Candidates for the Final must be registered with the College still, have either passed the Primary or been accepted as exempt (for example having passed the Diploma of the European Academy of Anaesthesiology or the Fellowship exams of various foreign colleges or their equivalents), have been a specialist registrar or recognised trainee equivalent for at least 6 months and had a minimum of 30 months' satisfactory approved anaesthetic training. Candidates for both parts have to get signatures from various lofty individuals in their departments to confirm they are who they say they are; they also have to part with considerable amounts of cash for the privilege of sitting the exams. One thing to make certain of when planning to sit the exam is that you can meet the practical requirements and deadline for applications. Details of these and the fee required may be obtained from your College Tutor or the College itself.

One criticism of candidates who fail is that many of them take the exam when they are not really ready, just to try it out because somehow they feel it is expected of them. This should not happen if individuals follow the Royal College guidelines and consult their College Tutor. Only 4 attempts at the Primary and 6 at the Final exams are allowed; in the good old days there was no limit and there are anaesthetists around who were legends in their own lifetime as having sat one part or other ten, fifteen or even more times. Most of these underground heroes were and are actually very good anaesthetists; at the very least they demonstrated amazing perserverence and were held in awe by lesser mortals if only for the fact that they must have singlehandedly funded a CEPOD report each. Now that a set number of attempts are allowed, the examiners hope that candidates will only take the exam when they are ready and be better prepared when they do so.

Structure of the exam

The make-up of both parts has changed already since conception, and is likely to undergo further fine-tuning as their performance is monitored. The actual subjects covered are described in Chapter 2, whilst this chapter considers the structure and scope of the exams themselves. Each part is administered by a separate group of examiners and there are working parties who set the questions for each section within each part.

Primary
The Primary exam consists of three sections: the MCQ paper, the vivas and the OSCEs (the last two together constitute the 'oral' part of the exam). When the modern Primary was first held, all candidates automatically sat all three parts, but since the start of 1998 only those who have a chance of passing the whole exam, go on to sit the orals. This has obvious advantages to both examiners and candidates in terms of not wasting people's time, and the initial 'lead in' period was to allow more experience with the new exam's format to be accrued.

The Primary MCQ paper covers pharmacology, physiology, biochemistry, physics and clinical measurement, clinical anaesthesia and basic statistics. The OSCEs cover various aspects of clinical practice and the vivas cover the same subjects as the MCQ paper. Thus the Primary exam has incorporated the old parts I and II exams; this fact has been forgotten by a number of Primary candidates who have realised too late that the exam is more than just a clinical one and contains a lot of basic science too. This basic science angle is somewhat at odds with the clinical emphasis of the Primary discussed in the next paragraph, and is perhaps one reason why the Primary exam and its scope have caused a fair amount of difficulty with candidates and even the odd examiner too.

The Primary tests 'understanding of the fundamentals of clinical anaesthetic practice including equipment and resuscitation; ... knowledge of the fundamental principles of anatomy, physiology, pharmacology, physics, clinical measurement and statistics as is appropriate for the discipline of anaesthesia; (and) ... skills and attitudes appropriate to the above level of training'. As you can see, this definition is a bit woolly but it serves to set the scene for what is required of you. The College acknowledges that after 1–1 ½ years' anaesthesia, many candidates will not have deep knowledge of every subject. The exam is designed to discriminate between candidates who are good and those who are poor, and not between those who are good and those who are excellent. It thus functions as a screening tool to help identify junior doctors who perhaps shouldn't be thinking of careers in anaesthetics, before they get on to the SpR wagon train and can't get off. In fact, since clinical medicine makes up such a large part of clinical anaesthesia, the Primary FRCA may also help to identify those who perhaps may not be suited to medicine itself. The Primary exam features a lot of fairly basic medicine, and may thus be seen as providing a service in protecting patients at a very basic level, not just as a hurdle to be jumped.

Final

The Final is concerned with the basic science and practice of clinical anaesthesia, intensive care and pain, and is thus intended as a test of basic competence and safety of anaesthetists who are committed to their specialty. Candidates should have 'a knowledge of medicine and surgery appropriate to the practice' of the above specialties and the 'ability to apply that knowledge' in these 'broad fields... covered during training for this examination' (as if the blurb for the Primary wasn't woolly enough). To give the College credit, it's difficult to define an exam accurately, let alone two exams, and the fact that these kind of statements exist at all is a major advance. Again, it is ackowledged that whilst knowledge of the principles of specialised areas of training is required, details are not.

The Final exam also consists of three sections, but two of them are in the written part (the MCQ and SAQ papers) and one in the oral part (the vivas). The written part must be passed in order to sit the oral.

The Final MCQ paper covers medicine, surgery, applied basic sciences, clinical measurement, intensive care, clinical anaesthesia and pain management. The SAQ paper covers clinical anaesthetic topics and the vivas cover clinical anaesthesia and applied basic sciences.

About 95% of candidates who passed the old FRCA took four tries or fewer to achieve success, hence the number of attempts allowed as the maximum under current College guidelines. Although older generations may look back fondly at pass rates in single figures, current pass rates are in the order of 40–50% (and yes, women candidates do slightly better than men).

The College allows observers to attend the the orals of either part of the exam, partly to demonstrate the open nature of the exam; partly to aid the training of future candidates; and partly to encourage Fellows to apply to become examiners. Potential observers must be either College Council members, College Tutors, examiners-elect, consultant Fellows (previously of five years' standing), senior representatives of other august bodies, or others of comparable status with these requirements. Observers are made very welcome at the exam and are allowed to sit in on several tables each and ask questions of the examiners, although they are not allowed to get involved in any candidate's actual performance. Up to eight are allowed on any one day and they are well looked after; at the very least, it's a good quality free lunch so you should tell your seniors that it's worth doing if they haven't already done so.

Marking

The same basic method of marking is used for all parts of both exams, based on a fairly narrow range of possible marks.

- 0 Veto: the candidate is absent (or their answer is) and therefore cannot score at all.
- 1 The candidate has failed poorly.
- 1+ The candidate has failed, although only just; it is still possible to pass the exam depending on the candidate's marks in other questions (see below).
- 2 The candidate has passed.
- 2+ This score is only given if the candidate is being considered for a prize, for which a 2+ in every part of the exam at the first sitting is required.

If a 1 is scored in any question, the candidate has failed that part of the exam however well he or she performs on other questions; he or she is allowed to score a single 1+ and still pass if all other questions receive marks of 2. A mark of 2+ cannot offset a mark of 1 elsewhere. Some of the subtleties of marking individual parts of the exams are discussed in the appropriate chapters, but the above scheme applies to all parts.

One consequence of this 'close marking' scheme is that assuming you turn up and you're not prize material, there are only three marks you can get: 1, 1+ or 2 (representing fail, bare fail and pass respectively). The most basic of answers should therefore get you at least into the upper 1+ range (excluding MCQs); it is that last 'push' which is so often sorely lacking and yet quite achievable with some solid thought and streetwise preparation.

All parts of the exams and their answers are subject to careful scrutiny in order to reject questions that are too easy or too difficult (e.g. every candidate passes or fails them respecively), whilst retaining for further use those questions which can identify the good candidates from those who fail the whole exam (i.e. good discriminatory questions). This is equally true of the oral parts of the exam and even the performance of individual examiners, although it is easiest and most intuitively obvious with the MCQ paper.

Exam theory

Much has been written about which qualities can or should be tested by an exam, and to be honest, it's pretty boring stuff. Basic knowledge, practical skills, problem-solving and attitudes are reasonably straightforward, but when it comes to self-organisation, personal growth, different types of knowledge (core, focused and behaviour justification) and so on, my eyes start to glaze, I have to admit. Similarly, performance of examiners comes in for the same sort of scrutiny and analysis, for example classifying examiners' errors and identifying particular aspects of the interpersonal interaction between candidate and examiner as potential sources of inconsistency. That last sentence alone caused significant eye-glazing on my part, and this might be a good opportunity to reassure you that there will be little, if any, theoretical psychology or related waffling in the ensuing pages.

My exam theory is simple: success is 40% knowledge; 60% technique and organisation of that knowledge; and a variable amount (0–100%) of luck. Books on anaesthesia and astrology may help with the first and last of these three components respectively; it is the second at which this book is directed.

Revision

Make no mistake, you've got to get your head down and prepare yourself for the exam. Remember, the myth of the Ideal Student is largely just that, a myth. Also, there are strict rules about what exam candidates tell each other, and these rules have been handed down through the generations since time immemorial. Thus, whilst everyone may tell you they are working really hard in the 3–6 months leading up to an exam, when the exam actually approaches, everyone denies that they are doing any work at all. This is partly an external manifestation of the inner turmoil candidates face, and partly a not-very-subtle way of preparing for possible failure (if only I'd worked harder ...).

The task ahead

To prepare for the exam, you need to acquire or consolidate a number of things:

- Knowledge: pretty obvious on the face of it, but suprisingly often overlooked.
- Practical skills: you may be tested on these in action, or simply by your ability to describe how you do certain procedures.
- Problem-solving: the ability to interpret information and suggest courses of action is one thing we tend to be groomed towards during our long undergraduate and post-graduate training, and we rely on this every time we face a patient. However, streamlining this into an exam setting

can be difficult although it may be a good exercise for future clinical application.

- Exam technique: the ability to persuade the examiners how fantastic you really are underneath that quivering, blubbering mess that faces them. Much of this is related to the previous point.
- Attitudes: harder to define; basically you have to be able to demonstrate that you are a caring, sensitive but decisive sort of person, who can make the appropriate decisions in the context of the whole patient. The best source of inspiration for this is usually your own department and its members (who may influence you either positively or negatively in this regard).

There are a few encouraging thoughts which you should bear in mind and repeat to yourself at intervals throughout the whole business of preparation for and sitting of the exams. First, you **can** do it; just look around at who else has in the past. Second, the examiners are humans too; imagine them at home, doing the weeding, having a bath, or whatever else you do at home (try not to spend too much time on this one). Third, in a perverse sort of way (as if the previous one wasn't perverse enough), it's quite nice being knowledgeable about what you're doing; it makes you think about your day-to-day anaesthetic practice and may actually be making you a better anaesthetist. Finally, you **can** do it.

Getting going

One of the hardest parts of revising is starting. Faced with an overwhelming range of topics to learn, it is tempting to fall back on simple denial and wait 'just another week' before starting. This is dangerous and you must have a method not only for getting going, but also for picking up speed. People will do the most extraordinary things to fool themselves they are 'revising' without actually doing anything of the sort. Compiling complicated three-dimensional revision timetables with six colours can take several hours of hard work (I speak from experience) and creates the right impression of your dedication and toil amongst your friends and family, but is probably a little unnecessary. I've known colleagues spend fortunes buying every single textbook they can find, filling all their available shelf space and generating hours of happy and comforting reorganising of their personal libraries. This is inappropriate: there is rarely time to read all those books and carrying around pristine tomes which have obviously been untouched since their purchase does little for the studious impression you are trying to make on others and yourself.

As in the above examples, the basic delusion to which we all fall prey is that there can be any real alternative to hard work, which there isn't. You can of course just launch into revising by blitzing a subject and then moving on to another, and so on, but most people I speak to find this hard to do and rather inefficient in terms of usage of time, since it offers no overall structure or indication of progress. There are, though, a number of useful ways in which you can get into the frame of things.

- Draw up a revision plan, but sensibly. This can be used as a guide for the entire period leading up to the exam and is well worth doing (see below).
- Make a conscious effort to read those journals you've been avoiding: you're going to have to read them at some point so you might as well start now. Setting a target of, say, one issue per day of any anaesthetic journal provides a relatively easily attainable task which will also be useful to you. Nobody expects you to be able to quote hundreds of recent papers to support particular points, especially for the Primary, but flicking through a journal is a fairly good way of trying to stimulate a modicum of interest (a tip: avoid any paper that involves animals, especially small furry ones, or measurement of plasma levels of anything).
- A method which I personally favour is to start compiling a list of those vital statistics beloved of anaesthetic exams: drug details and doses, physical data relating to volatile agents, classic physics and physiology formulae, statistical and pharmacological definitions, composition of i.v. fluids, physiological data, and so on. You'll find that the list

grows as you look around for more things to include (you never know, it might one day be publishable as a textbook). This list can become a major tool in your revision programme (see later), and putting it together is a good way of getting yourself to think about the various topics relatively easily.

- Take a look at the protocols and guidelines that exist in your department, and make sure you are familiar with the subjects covered.
- An obvious step is to go on a course (see later). There are several of these, and they are often timed around the exams. Part of their benefit is derived from mingling with others in a similar position, and swapping tips. However, courses are notorious for giving a false sense of revision security ('How's the revising going?' 'Fine thanks, I'm going on a course').

With all these methods of getting going and also with the main revision itself, it is important not to be too ambitious with your aims, since allowing yourself to slip can be very demoralising as the amount of work required to 'catch up' increases in front of your eyes. Having made your plans and set your targets, though, it is vital that you be absolutely rigid with sticking to them. If you are one of those few fortunate people who can sail through exams by simply reading around haphazardly, you will ignore this advice, but most of us need some sort of framework to which to cling. In a similar way to dieting, having and sticking to a plan seems to work much better than playing it by ear. As with dieting, discipline is vital (unlike dieting, nobody publishes your photograph in magazines when you're successful).

Your life at home and at work also needs organising, as already mentioned. You need time, space, understanding, support, regular cups of coffee and the odd neck massage. Few of us manage to obtain all of these ever, let alone before an exam, but this could be your best chance yet.

Planning your revision

Most experienced exam teachers advise some sort of plan for revision, partly to ensure you cover all the required ground, partly to pace yourself and partly to highlight your progress so far and thus inspire a sense of achievement and confidence. Until recently, the 'required ground' was a rather nebulous concept but the publication of the FRCA Syllabus has made it much easier to know your enemy. On the down side, it means you only have yourself to blame if you miss out a bit and get asked about it on the day.

The first task in drawing up a revision plan is to decide when to start. The choice must vary depending on the individual; you should know by now whether 2, 3 or 6 months suits you for exams generally. You don't want to peak too early but on the other hand it would be nice to peak at some point. I'd suggest a total of 4–6 months with a lead-in period of about 2–3 months, allowing a good 3 months for 'quality' revision.

What to cover

The subjects themselves are best tackled by listing the major subject headings and the topics within them. The FRCA Syllabus will be very helpful here as it gives fairly detailed guidance on most topics, and you must get a copy and study it well. The Syllabus headings are:

Primary

- Anaesthesia and resuscitation
- Anatomy
- Physiology and biochemistry
- Pharmacology
- Physics and clinical measurement
- Basic statistics
- Skills

Final

- Anaesthesia
- Applied anatomy
- Applied physiology
- Applied clinical pharmacology
- Clinical measurement
- Intensive care medicine
- Pain management

Although the topics listed under each heading are fairly comprehensive, the headings themselves are rather broad. It may be worthwhile breaking them down into more manageable chunks; for example:

- Anatomy
- Regional techniques
- Physiology
- Pharmacology
- Physics/clinical measurement/equipment
- General medicine/intensive care
- Obstetrics/paediatrics
- Pain/resuscitation
- Complications
- Anaesthetic management of ...
- Other

Some of these headings may not obviously go together (e.g. pain and resuscitation) but I have grouped them to form blocks of roughly similar size, which is useful when going through the various headings. Although the two parts of the exam differ in their coverage, both will include topics from the above list, even if only briefly for the Primary.

The last three headings merit special comment. So many exam questions relate to complications of anaesthesia, and complications are so important in clinical practice, that a separate block of topics seems appropriate. The 'Anaesthetic management of ...' heading is a very useful one and would include the type of question 'how would you manage a patient with [insert condition here] who is having a [insert procedure here]'. There are a number of 'classic' conditions from which to choose and they can all be listed under this heading (see later). The procedure is usually abdominal or trauma surgery, or surgery specific to the patient's condition. The question can also be directed at the anaesthetic management of routine cases (e.g. 'How would you anaesthetise for a total hip replacement?') so standard procedures also can be listed here. The 'Other' heading refers to those extra topics that always crop up: official reports, safety hazard bulletins, current items in the news, etc. Many will be more appropriate to the viva than to the written parts of the exam but should be listed here anyway.

Sample topics are shown in the Appendix, which is an amalgam of the FRCA Syllabus and my own topic list, lovingly collected over the years. Whereas the Syllabus describes topics in rather broad terms, I've included specific scenarios and cases which can be used to practise individual answers. You will see that I have distributed topics relating to specialist surgery throughout the other headings, and have deliberately mixed up some of the topics within each heading to make life a little more interesting (for example, textbooks tend to bore you first with basic sciences before you get to the clinical nitty gritty). Needless to say, you can arrange the topics as you wish; you can add your own topics as they occur to you or as they become trendy. You may of course find that you prefer the broad heading layout of the FRCA Syllabus itself rather than my more broken-down lists, or you may find that both can be used together. Please note that I have not attempted to provide any actual answers to questions: if you were looking for a book of practice exam questions I'm afraid this isn't it.

The actual content of the subject lists will of course vary according to the part of the exam being sat, and also from year to year (or as often as the FRCA Syllabus is updated) as subjects become lower- or higher-profile. In addition, there may be overlap, e.g. epidural analgesia for labour may be listed under 'Regional anaesthesia' or 'Obstetric anaesthesia'. For really important subjects such as epidurals in labour, this is actually a good way of ensuring you go through the topic thoroughly by having you go through it more than once.

From the topic list in the Appendix or Syllabus (or your own if you prefer), you can draw up a revision plan by putting the headings down the left-hand column and listing the topics in columns, along the lines of the sample revision plan (part, at least) shown in Box 2.1. This way you can see at a glance all the topics you have yet to cover or have already covered, and is probably easier to manage than keeping page after page of lists to look through. You can list the topics in several short columns as done here or a few, very long ones.

Box 2.1 Part of a revision plan.

Anatomy	Carotid arteries Cervical spine	Internal jugular and subclavian veins
Regional anaesthesia	Lumbar epidurals Spinals	Thoracic and cervical epidurals
Physiology	Function of lungs, liver	Control of BP Cardiac cycle
Pharmacology	Drugs which lower BP	Side-effects of drugs Interactions
Physics, Measurement, Equipment	Measurement of volatile agents	Measurement of body fluids
Medicine, ICU	TPN	IPPV and its modes
Obstetrics, Paediatrics	Physiological effects of pregnancy	Premedication in children
Pain, CPR	Measurement of pain Pain pathways	Basic, advanced CPR
Complications	Post-operative confusion	Post-operative jaundice
Anaesthetic management of ...	Dystrophia myotonica Marfan's	Myasthenia gravis Carcinoid
Other	Pre-operative investigations	ASA scoring system Consent

Finally, you shouldn't forget specific parts of the exam such as the MCQ and SAQ papers, etc. Thus, as well as plodding through the topics in your revision plan as discussed below, you should also earmark time for practising these techniques. You can do this by adding an extra row to your plan after the 'Other' heading in Box 2.1, marked 'MCQ/SAQ' or suchlike. When you come to this row, spend the allotted time practising MCQs/SAQs, and so on. Once the written part of the exam has been taken, this extra heading can be retitled 'Viva/ OSCE' if you wish (obviously there is no point spending time at this point in the proceedings practising MCQs, for example), although I'd suggest deleting the heading altogether and just changing your approach to the subjects themselves (see specific chapters). In general, there's little point revising specifically for the oral part until the written part is out of the way; you've got to get through the written part to have a chance at the orals anyway and so you must give the written paper priority at this stage. Also, the revision you do for the written exam will serve you well for the orals, whereas the opposite is less true. Finally, you will have had enough of revision anyway by the time you start revising for the orals, and starting a different approach after the written exam might just help inject a little extra spice into the process, although I accept this is a long shot.

How to cover the topics

Once you have a list of the subjects to be covered, there are three main ways of going through them.

1 Bulldozing: covering all aspects of an area and its related topics. For example, you could go through the anatomy of the heart, its physiology, relevant pharmacology, management of patients with heart disease, etc. An alternative version is to plough through **all** the physiology subjects (i.e. all systems), then go through **all** the pharmacology, etc. Both these approaches allow you to 'do' a subject thoroughly and also follow natural connections between related topics. However, it can be rather dull spending a long period on just one major topic (let's be honest, a lot of it is hardly gripping stuff). Also, the feeling of being stuck in one area and never getting around to the others can be a little worrying as the weeks go by.

2 Random scatter: zipping from one topic to another with no overall pattern. This is probably the best way of not getting stuck in a rut but has the danger of leaving out unpopular topics unless you force yourself to be truly random.

3 Lawnmowing: moving down the major subject headings in a set order. For example, for the part of a revision plan shown in Box 2.1 which is taken from the Appendix, this would entail revising an anatomy topic first, then a regional anaesthesia one, then physiology, then pharmacology, physics, etc. When you reach the end, start again with anatomy, and so on. I personally prefer this method as it provides a reasonable amount of variety but also gives a degree of

continuity since you can pass down the plan fairly quickly and rejoin a major subject where you left off last time.

With all these methods, it is important to chart your progress by marking those topics you've covered, e.g. by putting a tick or red bullet mark next to the topic. This provides visual encouragement that you are making progress and gives an indication of how often you've covered each topic. This is especially useful for particular 'hot' topics that you know you must cover well, i.e. more than once, such as failed intubation drill, CPR, etc., or those topics you've predicted as likely to come up, as discussed below.

Question spotting

When the essays were a major part of the exams, predicting questions was an easier task than it is now, since there was a degree of consistency from year to year and only five or six questions for each exam. With the introduction of the new short-answer format, there is less certainty about their content, and a pattern has yet to emerge. Still, the sort of topics chosen is likely to remain similar to those of the old exam, and it should be possible to identify those topics especially likely to appear. For example, Box 2.2 shows the last 5 years' topics for the Part III/Final exam (the format of the old Part I/new Primary has changed more than that of the Part III/Final, making it harder to spot questions; also, the Primary written paper now consists of MCQs only). Use the space for 1998 and the margin for subsequent papers (ask colleagues or fill them in yourself, although I hope you won't have too many personal exposures to the exam yourself). Current trendy subjects or new techniques usually take a year or so to filter through into the written parts of the exam, but can also be 'spotted' to some extent. Of course, whilst question-spotting is fun and may indicate which areas require particular attention, you cannot afford to miss out major topics since you could legitimately be asked about anything included in the Syllabus.

Box 2.2 Question subjects for the recent Part III/Final FRCA written exams in recent years. NB there may be overlap between headings, e.g. all question on regional techniques will include anatomy and often complications.

Year	1993	1994	1995	1996	1997	1998
Anatomy		Pleura and interpleural analgesia		Trachea and bronchi	Internal jugular vein + cannulation	
Regional anaesthesia	Eye blocks Intercostal block	Brachial plexus blocks	Stellate ganglion For hand surgery	For day-case knee surgery Epidurals Axillary block	Spinal for TURP	
Physiology						
Pharmacology	Place of N_2O	Hypokalaemia			Antihypertensives	
Physics/ measurement/ equipment	Measurement of blood gases Measurement of temperature	Capnography LMA Electrical hazards	Measurement of volatile agents Measurement of cardiac output on ICU Ventilation techniques	Radial artery BP measurement	Monitoring in the MRI scanner Statistical comparison of two sets of data	
Medicine/ICU	Transport of critically-ill patients Assessment of nutrition	Head injury ARDS	Cardiac output monitoring Chest trauma	Organ retrieval Acute head injury Status asthmaticus	Pulmonary artery catheters Indications for tracheostomy Management of hypertension on ICU Head injury–factors exacerbating primary brain damage Venous thrombosis–risk factors + prevention	

Box 2.2 *continued*

Year	1993	1994	1995	1996	1997	1998
Obstetrics/ Paediatrics	6-week-old for pyloric stenosis Caesarean section for PET	Massive obstetric haemorrhage	3-year-old with stridor 3-month-old for day case hernia Hypotension after Caesarean section	Spinal surgery Acute hypoxaemia after Caesarean section	Paediatric post-operative analgesia Management of dural tap Reduction in maternal mortality	
Pain/CPR	Post-operative pain; PCA vs epidural Management of asystole			PCA Reflex sympathetic dystrophy	Post-laparotomy analgesia Causes, effects and treatment of neurogenic pain	
Complications	Post-operative nausea and vomiting Intra-operative heat loss	Arrhythmias Awareness Fat embolism Problems in recovery Electrical hazards	Intra-operative MH Arrhythmias	Perioperative MI Intra-arterial thiopentone Aspiration pneumonitis Collapse in the dental chair (LA) Awareness Complications of epidurals	Of blood transfusion Effect of age on morbidity and mortality of lithotomy + head-down tilt following CABG	

Box 2.2 *continued*

Year	1993	1994	1995	1996	1997	1998
Anaesthetic management of....	Facial trauma	Phaeochromo-cytoma ENT laser surgery Aortic aneursym	History of bleeding for major surgery Carotid endarterectomy Chronic renal failure for fistula Myasthenia gravis for laparotomy Facial trauma	Bronchoscopy 12-year-old for kyphoscoliosis surgery Paraplegic for laparotomy Pericardectomy for constrictive pericarditis	Patient with pacemaker Fractured ankle + head injury Fractured neck of femur + atrial fibrillation Heroin addict Ischaemic heart disease COAD for TURP	
Other	Preoxygenation Sedation				GA and the eye	

What to do when and when to do what

So now you have a list of topics to revise and a plan for how to go through them. Next, you have to pace your progress to ensure you cover the whole ground. If you give yourself enough time (I'd suggest 3 months as a minimum), it should be possible not only to go through the complete plan, but to do so several times. This is where revising a topic already marked from a previous run-through is particularly satisfying, as well as being more efficient in terms of retention. If you start out with an open mind and see how far you get in the first week or two, or alternatively how long it takes you to get through say, 10–20 individual topics, you should be able to concentrate on slowing down or speeding up as appropriate. I should aim at going through the entire list at least twice, and more often if possible. Of course, nearer the time it would probably be worth leaving out the more obscure topics and concentrating on the more certain ones.

Revision methods

Structured revision

Once you've cleared the social decks, arranged psychological support, enlisted friends, family and colleagues, promised yourself specific treats (or beatings) to spur you on and drawn up a plan for the next several months, it's time to sit down and go through the material. To do this you must have time on your own, free of distractions; for example reading a chapter of a textbook whilst watching *Eastenders* is as useful as reading the back of a cereal packet (or as generally useful as ...well, watching *Eastenders*). You must give yourself an allotted time every day for proper revision. This is best measured in hours and I'd suggest 1–2 hour blocks as the minimum base unit; most people find less than an hour is simply too short a period to allow any constructive revision (although beware the temptation to divide the evening into 45 minute slots which you then don't use because you can't do anything in only 45 minutes. In fact, you can always fill a short slot by drawing and redrawing a diagram or two). Thus for example your average evening could be divided into two 2 hour sessions with a break in between. It's important to set yourself the task in advance (e.g. deciding on the way home how many hours you'll do that evening) because you can then plan your evening around the revision sessions. As already mentioned, you should be realistic in setting your targets and not be too ambitious (after all, you are an anaesthetist, not a surgeon), and you should be absolutely determined to achieve however many sessions you have set yourself. The 'I'll just start and see how it goes' approach generally doesn't work as well and is not as good for charting your progress. Setting yourself a target and achieving it does great things for your confidence, too, but try to resist the temptation of celebrating by having the next week off. Having said that, you may need to bribe yourself with various rewards for accomplishing the set task(s) of the day, especially at the beginning. However, if you do this you **must** be strict and only grant yourself the prize if you achieve the goal.

Planned breaks are an important part of the revision process. Making yourself a drink (or having one made for you) is a good way to break up a long tedious evening, as long as you limit the time used up (5–10 minutes should suffice) and the alcohol intake. During this allotted time, it's worth making the conscious effort to relax and clear your mind. Music is a particularly good tool for distracting the troubled mind from academic matters; twanging a guitar or other instrument may do wonders for you, if not for your family/flatmates/neighbours. Another method is to clap on some headphones and play a favourite piece of music, preferably very loudly. After experimenting with different musical styles, you'll find the one which releases most tension and clears the mind best (for what it's worth, mine has been 'Rocky Mountain Way' by Joe Walsh ever since my schooldays, but yours could be anything from classic opera to the theme from *Teletubbies*).

Once it comes down to the subjects themselves, there are many ways of going through them (more specific advice is offered in the chapters relating to specific parts of the exam).

Reading books
Books are invaluable sources of information, largely because someone else has taken the trouble to sift out the rubbish and present the useful material in (you hope) a user-friendly way. However, reading can take up a lot of time and be done whilst you are half-asleep with very little benefit to you. (How often have you read a whole page only to realise you haven't taken in a single word?) Also, just because a book exists does not guarantee that it is written well or even that it is correct. Finally, beware the dangers of having too many books: you may not be able to carry them all, let alone read them all. In addition, the more authorities you consult, the more different opinions you obtain. None the less, books are a very useful adjunct to revision if used alongside other methods.

There is an increasing number of anaesthestic textbooks from which to choose; for help in selection consult fellow trainees. Ideally, borrow one or two from friends or a library, and look up a few sample topics in each to see how they compare. For the exams with their pressures of limited time, I have always favoured short and concise texts over more verbose ones, but others may like the feel and style of the larger authoritative books.

Reading journals
You must do this, but don't let it interfere with your revision plan as outlined above. As a primary source of information, journals probably represent a rather inefficient way of spending your blocks of revision time, unless the article concerned is a good review of a not too esoteric subject. You're probably better off collecting good references from books, reviews, your colleagues or your own browsing, and going through the articles at other times (see bath-time revision, below). In general, of the most accessible journals, I have found that the editorials and reviews in the *British Journal of Anaesthesia*, *Anaesthesia*, the *Canadian Journal of Anaesthesia* and *Anaesthesia & Intensive Care* are the most user-friendly, with those in *Anesthesia & Analgesia* and *Anesthesiology* usually more complex but often worth a look if you have time. There are also specific review-type journals (e.g. *Current Opinions in Anesthesiology* and *Current Anaesthesia*

& Critical Care): these have their own enthusiastic followers but I'd recommend that you borrow an issue or two to look at before subscribing to see if they suit you. *Current Opinions* has more of a review-of-the-last-year approach so may be less useful for general reviews. Remember, the more material you have to read, the more material you have to read.

With these journals, you should at least flick through the last 2–3 years' worth to see if anything catches your eye. I'd suggest doing this even for the Primary, although it is more important you do this for the Final. It is probably less worthwhile going through more general medical journals, more specific anaesthetic ones or even the intensive care ones, unless you have a specific paper to look up.

Note taking

I was never any good at this, but it was always a very popular method of revising amongst my colleagues. Having a large and comprehensive series of authoritative notes on the whole syllabus is certainly attractive, but by the time you've finished the task, you've got another wad of paperwork to read and used up a large proportion of your time. Borrowing others' notes always seemed daft to me; everyone has a different way of making notes and a different emphasis. For example, nobody ever asked to borrow mine more than once because my notes consisted of headings only and were full of little abbreviations that no-one else could understand.

Writing cue cards

Although similar to note taking, this seems more efficient in terms of use of time, since all you need to write on each card are the bare essentials for each topic (in fact, this is the way some people take notes anyway). Each term written then acts as a prompt rather than a source of information in its own right. This style of annotating goes well with writing essay plans.

Writing essay plans

Although the essays hated and feared by generations of anaesthetists are no more, the skeletons on which they were constructed remain a useful way of covering a subject. In fact, the humble essay plan has emerged as one of the best ways of preparing answers for SAQs as well as the orals, since it allows you to practice angling a response towards a directed question. Many questions fall into groups of similar types, and can be tackled in similar ways (Box 2.3). For example, an answer can be put together for any of the topics in the Appendix: each plan should be relatively short and logically set out with a beginning, middle and end as shown. Many 'Causes of...' questions can be approached using a standard list of general causes of disease or symptoms. At medical school this was always referred to as the 'Surgical Sieve' but I could never understand why the surgeons claimed ownership. Perhaps it reflected their fascination with metal objects or perhaps it was an ironic reminder of the high esteem with which all other specialties regard surgeons' grasp of internal medicine. Either way, the sieve is a very useful tool on which to fall back, both academically and clinically. You may well have your own by now; mine has the mnemonic TINVINEMIDIP which is hardly inspiring but it is useful (Box 2.4). I've had this ridiculous mnemonic for about 20 years now but still use it if faced with an unusual clinical situation when I want to be sure I've thought of everything. There may be considerable overlap between causes but the list will cover most things. Try it for coma, vomiting, etc.

The plans themselves should follow a similar pattern: each should have a title, beginning, middle and end, with lots of underlining and subheadings to emphasise the structure of the answer. The title helps you remember how the answer should be pitched. Wherever possible, concentrate on common points, not rare ones. Try to think in headings rather than small print (I find it helpful to imagine chapters in a book on the subject rather than individual pages). Use arrows to link different parts of the plan, add afterthoughts or structure your answer into a logical order: some samples are shown in Figure 2.1.

The advantage of using essay plans as a form of revision is that each plan only takes a short time, so it is possible to get through a lot of topics in a fixed revision session. Also, having first gone through a topic in its entirety, you can then set yourself a specific 'exammy' approach to the topic, e.g.

Box 2.3 Examples of essay plans as a means of revising a subject.

a) **Question:**	How would you manage a patient with condition x for operation y?
Essay plan:	Introduction: Incidence/background to condition x Effects of condition x on pre-existing state Effects of anaesthesia/surgery on condition x Special requirements of operation y
	Pre-operative: Assess as for any procedure but especially for aspects discussed above Pre-operative treatment/premedication
	Per-operative: Check equipment/monitoring/staff Induction/maintenance/recovery Fluids/position/other
	Post-operative: Analgesia/special care/fluids
b) **Question:**	What are the problems of operation y?
Essay plan:	Introduction: incidence of operation y and its complications
	Patients: age/predisposing conditions
	Position: e.g. lithotomy, prone, etc.
	Procedure: any special maneouvres e.g. insufflation, cement, etc.
c) **Question:**	What are the causes of acute sympton z?
Essay plan:	(i) Approach via anatomy/physiology e.g. for dyspnoea, start at the face and work back to the lungs and thence to the respiratory centre.
	(ii) Approach via Surgical Sieve (see text+ Box 2.4).
d) **Question:**	What are the characteristics of the ideal ... agent?
Essay plan:	Manufacture/storage of drug
	Getting the drug to the patient: preparation/administration/physical properties
	Effects of the drug on the body (go through the systems)
	Quickly run through existing drugs to ensure you haven't missed out important effects.
e) **Question:**	How would you perform procedure x?
Essay plan:	Indications/contraindications
	Technique: patient's position; landmarks; approach; end-point; injection, etc.
	Effects of procedure (i.e. desirable ones)
	Complications (i.e. undesirable ones)

'What factors increase the likelihood of accidental dural tap' or 'How would you manage an accidental dural tap'. To get the most out of the technique, I would suggest writing a plan,

---

Box 2.4 Causes of everything; the 'Surgical Sieve'.

T – trauma
I – infective
N – neurological
V – vascular
I – inflammatory
N – neoplastic
E – endocrine
M – metabolic
I – iatrogenic
D – deficiency
I – idiopathic
P – psychological

---

then going through your notes, books or whatever to see what you missed out and then **re-doing** the plan again from scratch. This last part is very important, since it reinforces the changes you've made to your original answer. Just saying to yourself 'Oh yes, I forgot that bit' but not reinforcing it is unlikely to make you remember it next time. As a parting gesture to the topic concerned, and in order to prove to yourself that you know the subject, you can go through it once more verbally (see below) before moving on to the next topic. On successive passages through the topic list, you can vary the angle slightly to reduce monotony, for example using the two dural tap questions above.

Another useful thing to do with essay plans is to show them to each other and to respected elders in your department. For example, if three of you quickly write out a couple of plans on the same subject, you can compare them and see which bits each of you have missed out. Showing them to more senior anaesthetists may produce useful tips and identify omissions as well.

Practising giving a talk
This is similar to the essay plan method, but you have to imagine yourself talking to an audience instead of writing everything down. This method is especially important for the oral parts of the exam, but is also a useful alternative to the essay plan method for the written exam. The imaginary

Figure 2.1 Sample essay plans. (a) The effects of acute haemorrhage in a fit adult. (b) How to anaesthetise a rheumatoid arthritic patient for a hip replacment.

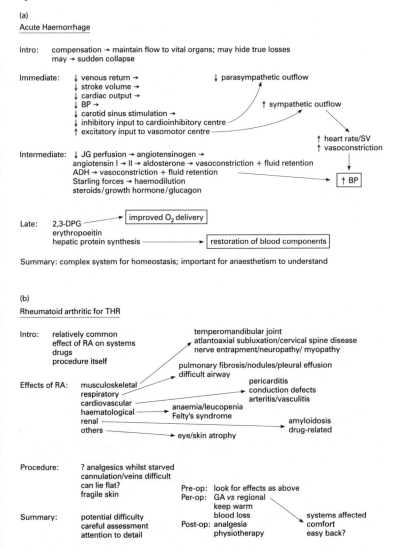

(a)

Acute Haemorrhage

Intro: compensation → maintain flow to vital organs; may hide true losses
             may → sudden collapse

Immediate: ↓ venous return →   ↓ parasympathetic outflow
             ↓ stroke volume →
             ↓ cardiac output →
             ↓ BP →   ↑ sympathetic outflow
             ↓ carotid sinus stimulation →
             ↓ inhibitory input to cardioinhibitory centre
             ↑ excitatory input to vasomotor centre
                                                        ↑ heart rate/SV
                                                        ↑ vasoconstriction

Intermediate: ↓ JG perfusion → angiotensinogen →
             angiotensin I → II → aldosterone → vasoconstriction + fluid retention
             ADH → vasoconstriction + fluid retention
             Starling forces → haemodilution   → ↑ BP
             steroids/growth hormone/glucagon

Late: 2,3-DPG ────→ improved O$_2$ delivery
         erythropoeitin
         hepatic protein synthesis ────────→ restoration of blood components

Summary: complex system for homeostasis; important for anaesthetism to understand

(b)

Rheumatoid arthritic for THR

Intro: relatively common
             effect of RA on systems   temperomandibular joint
             drugs   atlantoaxial subluxation/cervical spine disease
             procedure itself   nerve entrapment/neuropathy/ myopathy

                                             pulmonary fibrosis/nodules/pleural effusion
                                             difficult airway
Effects of RA: musculoskeletal   pericarditis
                respiratory   conduction defects
                cardiovascular   arteritis/vasculitis
                haematological   anaemia/leucopenia
                renal   Felty's syndrome   amyloidosis
                others   eye/skin atrophy   drug-related

Procedure: ? analgesics whilst starved
             cannulation/veins difficult
             can lie flat?   Pre-op: look for effects as above
             fragile skin   Per-op: GA vs regional
                                              keep warm
                                              blood loss   systems affected
Summary: potential difficulty   Post-op: analgesia   comfort
             careful assessment   physiotherapy   easy back?
             attention to detail

audience can be colleagues or examiners, but the 'do it once, look it up and do it again' technique should still apply. You should actually produce some noise so that you get used to the way your answers **sound**. I find a quiet whisper is adequate without scaring the children and still use this technique when practising lectures.

With the writing and speaking, what you're aiming to do is produce an answer to an imaginary question which you can then improve upon so that your answer next time will be better. Ideally, you will already have practised every single topic you get asked in the actual exam. Although this is unlikely, it's a good ideal for which to aim. It's certainly very obvious when questioning someone if they've never thought about that particular question before. Again, although particularly pertinent to the oral part, this may also come across in the SAQ; at the very least, practising the actual formation of a structured answer will save you time on the day.

It's important to reduce boredom by varying the approaches used; so you should consider using all of the above methods during your revision.

Courses

You should always try to get on to a course for both Primary and Final exams if you can. They'll often stimulate or scare you into revision, and you'll benefit from exposure to the thoughts and fears of others in similar situations. There's also something to be gained from meeting some of the big names you may have heard about and from their words of wisdom; and it's nice to see what they actually look like.

There are two problems with courses: which one to go on and when to go on it. The first question can only be answered by your colleagues or friends who have been to courses and can tell you about them. In practice, all courses are probably equally worthwhile but some may be more suited to you than others, although largely because of factors other than course content. For example, a day-release course over several months leading up to the exam or stopping a month or so before the exam will give you a welcome regular break from hospital work and give you more time to get yourself into the exam mood, whereas a 1–3 week intensive 'crammer' course suits some better by demanding and delivering more within a short period of time. Other factors to take into account include the course's cost, where it is held and your department's staffing arrangements. As to when to go on a course, there would be little point in going on a 1-week crammer 9 months before your exam, so you'll have to look around at what's available at the time. Most courses are pretty well publicised in the journals and via the College Tutors in each department. Don't forget to plan well in advance since you may have to negiotate study leave with other hopefuls in your department. It's probably worthwhile going to different centres for the Primary and Final courses if you can, since a single department that organises courses aimed at the two different parts of the exam will tend to use the same lecturers for many of the subjects, and it's nice to get a wider exposure. Whichever course you attend, make sure you talk to your fellow attendees, even if you're naturally a shy and retiring type like me. You'll get useful advice about questions, books, etc. and you'll keep coming across these same people throughout your career so you might as well start trying to remember their names now. However, beware the games that people play around exams (e.g. scaring the opposition, false rumours, etc.).

Bath-time revision

I use this term to include all unstructured but equally important types of revision. Coming up to the exam, you should consider each day and even each moment as a potential opportunity for revision. True, it makes you a dull companion but then excitement can wait until you've passed. There are a number of situations which can be turned into useful information-acquiring and consolidating exercises.

Operating theatre lists
Take time to examine every bit of equipment in your anaesthetic room, theatre, cupboard, etc. Imagine you are explaining to a new trainee what each one is, how it works, what all its markings mean, what sizes it comes in, what flow rates are

possible through it, what the pore size is, etc. Get someone to go through things with you if you don't know or can't find out. It's important to carry a notebook (or these days, a palm-top computer or organiser) at all times. Make sure you write down a list of things you need to look up every day, and make sure you do in fact look them up later. You can repeat the whole exercise with every drug in your drug cupboard. Similarly, every time you do a case, imagine you're answering a question on what complications may occur, which anaesthetic techniques are especially suitable, etc. If there's someone with you, get them involved. If they won't help, complain to your head of department or rota organiser (if they **are** the head of department or rota organiser, you're in trouble).

Odd minutes
Remember that list of useful numbers, equations etc. that you drew up when you started getting into an exam frame of mind? Keep the list with you always (e.g. in a diary or

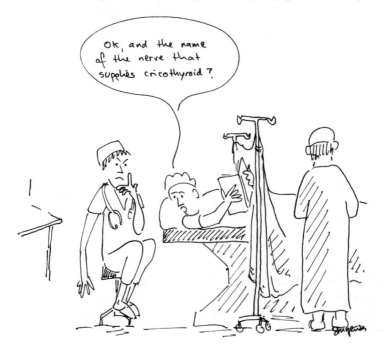

case) and force yourself to go through it **every** time you are alone in theatre. Test yourself on each item, writing out the correct answer each time you get it wrong. When you have to stop, mark the place and continue from there the next time. When you reach the end, start again at the beginning. You should be able to get through this list several times in the build-up to the exam. Although I admit this can be exceptionally tedious, it is a really useful way of learning those annoying little facts and figures. When you come to the exam itself, the last thing you need to do is to have to think about the boiling point of halothane or the ideal alveolar gas equation. If you know all these numbers by heart, it's really reassuring to be able to trot them out without any hesitation and also very impressive from the examiners' point of view. It also means you can avoid that awful situation of desperately trying to remember the boiling point of halothane with one half of your cerebral capacity whilst the other half is attempting to control the rapidly decompensating panic centre (located in the medulla just next to the nucleus pessimisticus). Although the 'Oh-God-I'm-going-to-fail-look-just-shut-up-and-think' syndrome is particularly acute during oral exams it can also occur during the written exams so this list-revision technique is well worth doing from the beginning. In addition, it allows you to drop impressive-looking numbers and formulae into written answers and handle related MCQs with greater confidence.

Diagrams
A similar approach can be used for diagrams. Make a list of those diagrams you **must** know but always forget, e.g. oxy-haemoglobin dissociation curve, brachial plexus, cross-section of the neck, etc. One by one, draw out the diagram from memory (such as it is), then look at the real version in a book or your notes, then draw it out again and so on until you can successfully reproduce it twice without making a mistake. Then, go on to the next one. Next time, carry on where you left off.

Practice answers
Whenever you have a spare moment, practise answering questions; you can make them up in your head or carry a list of 'topics du jour' around with you. This can easily be done on the way home, over meals, or even in the bath.

Look around
Preparing for an exam is also an excuse to be really nosy: keep going through your department's protocols, guidelines,

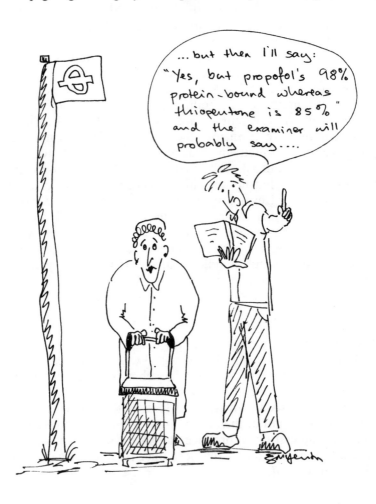

storage rooms, etc. and ask your senior colleagues (and drug reps!) about recent developments, reports, what's topical, and so on.

Collaboration

Team up with others and quiz each other, whether on practice MCQs, imaginary or real scenarios, etc. You might as well be sad and lonely people together.

Practical skills

Try hard to develop good practical skills: pay particular attention when watching others doing procedures and try to criticise them (to yourself). Be conscious of trying to achieve perfection when doing them yourself. For example, when you perform a regional block or invasive technique, describe to yourself the anatomy, technique, etc. as you do it. Developing good attitudes is harder but look around and watch/talk to your colleagues; identify the attributes that impress you and adopt them, whilst rejecting those that don't.

Drug names

Get used to referring drugs by their generic names, not their trade names. Saying 'Omnopon' or 'Zofran' in a written or spoken exam is like a red rag to a bull to most examiners and may even produce the same response. Write out the proper name every time you prescribe the drug or record its use on the anaesthetic chart.

Journals

Always carry a journal or two, or a good article, around with you. When you have a break and you can't face one of the above methods, go through them. By using your time employing different approaches, you're more likely to break the monotony and thus avoid boredom. Describe the interesting papers to your colleagues and get them to do the same back to you.

Summary

You will of course pick and chose what you want to do (if anything) from the above suggestions, but whatever you do decide upon, there are some general points which really must apply if you are to give yourself the best chance at going into the exams well prepared. Ensuring that you have general support at home and at work, planning your revision and dividing the tasks into attainable chunks, sticking to your plan like glue, building in breaks and treats, and above all changing the methods you use day-by-day or even session-by-session to maintain variety, will at the very least give a feeling of structure to your life at a time when stresses and pressures are building up to their worst. If you have found other techniques or strategies to be particularly useful for you, then you must stick with them – if you have particularly useful ones, please write and let me know.

The approaches described above should be applicable to both the Primary and the Final exams, and for all parts of the exams. However, tackling the more specific parts of the exams are discussed in subsequent chapters.

3

Multiple choice questions (MCQs)

MCQs are like a bad rash that keeps coming back to irritate you throughout your undergraduate and postgraduate career (or so I'm told). You probably will have ploughed through many MCQ papers by now, but few (if any) of us ever feel really comfortable with them, no matter how many we've done. Their popularity with examiners arises from many different properties: they're a relatively easy way of testing knowledge over a very wide range of topics; they can actually discriminate fairly well between candidates who eventually go on to do well and those who do badly; the questions can easily be stored in a database for subsequent use; good and bad questions can be identified by the mixture of responses obtained from a particular sitting and modified or left out next time (for example, if the top 50 candidates all do badly on one particular question despite their good performance in the rest of the paper, there is likely to be a problem with that question); and most importantly of all, they can be marked by a computer thus sparing examiners several hours of extra hassle which they can now spend arguing over the MCQ results the computer has produced.

The nature of the beast

For those of you who have been living on the Planet Zob for the last 10 years, there are different types of question. However, each has a 'stem' and five 'branches'; a stem is a statement or phrase and each branch may be true or false independently of the other branches. (There are some exams where only certain combinations of true/false answers are permitted, for example you answer 'A' if the first and third branches are correct; 'B' if the second, third but not the fourth are correct; 'C' if the third, fourth and fifth answers are incorrect and you had cornflakes for breakfast, and so on. Thankfully, this type of question, which can only have been devised under the influence of drugs, is not included in the FRCA exam.)

Some questions test knowledge of facts while others require some deduction or calculation. An example of the former might be 'Halothane may cause: (A) malignant hyperthermia; (B) uterine contraction; (C) bradycardia; etc. Obviously B is incorrect, since halothane causes uterine relaxation; stating the opposite of the truth is a common pattern in branches that are wrong, since it is actually quite difficult to make up an incorrect branch (you can never be sure that what you've made up is always the case. For example, i.v. lignocaine isn't exactly renowned for its ability to cause abdominal discomfort, but who's to say that it never does...). A deduction-type question might give some gas flow rates, the percentage of volatile agent dialled up on a vaporiser, and figures for atmospheric pressure. The branches might then say 'The partial pressure exerted by the volatile agent is x kPa', each branch giving a different value of x; you have to select one of these as correct (with the rest by definition being incorrect). Questions as clear cut as this are rare, since the examiners know that the wily candidate will simply mark each branch as incorrect, thus guaranteeing four plus marks and one minus mark (see below for details on marking). It's much more common now to find that the branches differ slightly in what they are saying, and that more than one can be right.

Both the Primary and Final exams have 90 MCQs to be answered in 3 h, divided up (approximately) as follows:

Primary: 30 pharmacology
         30 physiology and biochemistry
         30 physics and clinical measurement
Final: 20 medicine and surgery

20 applied basic science (including pharmacology and physiology

10 clinical measurement

20 intensive care

20 anaesthesia (including pain management)

Marking

Before talking about the overall strategy of answering the
MCQ paper, it's worth going over the marking system so
you can put things into context. A negative marking system
operates, whereby a correct answer to each branch of a question earns a mark but an incorrect one loses a mark; thus each
question carries a possible range of marks from -5 to $+5$. No
answer, of course, attracts no points. The MCQ paper therefore has the unique and rather dubious claim to fame of being
the only part of the exam in which it is possible to achieve a
mark of -100%.

Candidates are required to obtain a minimum mark in the
MCQ paper in order to sit the orals (previously this only
applied to the new Final whilst the new Primary was 'settling
in'). The pass mark is calculated as follows. All the candidates' actual scores (percentages) are added up and the mean
is calculated (the scores are virtually always normally distributed). The mean score is then tweaked acording to the scores
obtained from specific 'discriminator' questions, which indicate how the cohort of candidates as a whole has performed.
These discriminators are scattered throughout the paper and
have been found to predict overall performance closely.
Analysis of the discriminators enables the mean score to be
adjusted upward or downward by a small amount (usually
less than 1%) to compensate for the general level of the
cohort; thus for example an average candidate will not lose
out just because there happens to be an exceptionally good
bunch of candidates that year and the mean score is a bit
higher than usual. The adjusted score then becomes the
pass mark for that particular exam. Although the adjustment
may be a fraction of a percentage point, the correction may

affect a significant number of candidates since so many are clustered around the mean value. So, all those rumours about what the pass mark actually is for the MCQ don't really cover the whole story: the pass mark varies from sitting to sitting although it usually hovers around 50% (slightly under for the Primary; slightly over for the Final).

How do the actual percentages get converted to the 1, 1+, 2, 2+ scheme? Easy! Candidates scoring the pass mark receive the final MCQ mark of 2, with those achieving more than one standard deviation above, getting a 2+. Those within one standard deviation below the pass mark get a 1+, and those below one SD get a 1. Those who run screaming from the room after 30 s in a mass of pencils and gonks get a 0, and are 'eliminated', in the words of the College, along with those scoring a 1. Those getting a 1+ have a chance to pass if they get 2s in all other parts of the exam.

The rather complicated scheme described above is an amazing example of the efforts being made to mark the MCQs fairly and properly, and is a mixture of complex mathematical cal-

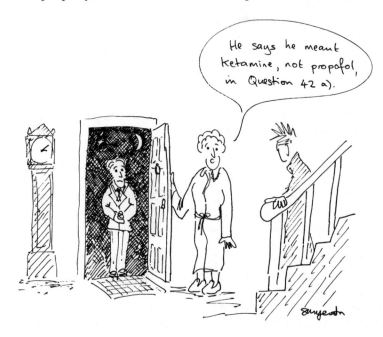

culation and pragmatism; the system works and is constantly under review.

Technique

The crucial aspect of answering MCQs is to make sure you read the question, as it's very easy to recognise a few key words in a question and jump to (erroneous) conclusions about the actual substance of the question. In particular, given that opposites are often inserted as described above, you can easily give the opposite answer by mistake. We're generally very good at recognising patterns without taking in the detail, hence the ease with which 'does' is mistaken for 'does not', 'hypo-' for 'hyper-', and so on. Similarly, it's easy to confuse similarly sounding drugs, such a chlorpromazine and chlorpropramide. These simple mistakes can be disastrous and result in a score of -5 instead of $+5$ for a particular question.

It often helps to read each branch as a continuation of the stem; for example if the stem is 'Atropine causes'; followed by (A) bradycardia; (B) sweating; (C) miosis, etc., then read to yourself 'Atropine causes bradycardia' when answering A; 'Atropine causes sweating' when answering B; 'Atropine causes miosis' when answering C, etc. Otherwise, it is easy to lose track of the thread of each question, especially if the question is a long one. Beware words like 'commonly', 'may', etc.; it can be hard to quantify just how frequent an event has to be in order to qualify for vague adjectives but it's also hard for the examiners to compile questions and they also have to make difficult decisions. If stuck as to whether the correct answer to a possibly ambiguous question is true or false, before leaving the question alone it may sometimes be worth thinking "what answer are they actually after?' For example, it is generally advised that propofol should be avoided in epileptic patients because it has been associated with post-operative convulsions and the Committee on the Safety of Medicines has issued a warning on this association. However, not all epileptic patients have problems after propofol and it has even been successfully used to **treat** status epilepticus. Thus the statement 'Propofol may be safely used in epileptic patients' is strictly speaking correct since it **may** be used safely. However, the question is more likely to be false than true since the examiners are more likely to be seeking your knowledge that propofol should probably not be used routinely in epileptics, than more detailed knowledge about complicated risk–benefit analysis of treatments in status epilepticus. This kind of ambiguity, which favours the less well-informed candidate over the know-all, should be rare given the ability of examiners to analyse the pattern of answers, detect bad questions and remove them.

Probably more than with any other part of the exam, there are countless theories circulating about the best strategic way to tackle MCQs, usually expressed with an accompanying slow indrawing of breath through pursed lips and a solemn shake of the head, akin to the response from a mechanic when asked to fix that rattling sound from behind the dashboard when you change rapidly from fourth gear to second. With luck, you will have evolved a successful strategy for yourself by now (and that is the important bit; what works for someone else may not be right for you), but I've found that most candidates are able to improve the marks they can achieve in practice papers (at least slightly) by changing the approach they take to MCQs, although I should state right now that if it doesn't work for you, it's not my fault.

Even if you feel relatively comfortable with MCQs, I would guess that you have probably have never formally tried different methods of actually answering them. I would strongly suggest that you try out the exercise described below – after all you have nothing to lose except a couple of hours. Having said that, making any improvement in your technique for answering MCQs requires a lot of discipline apart from a certain amount of experimentation. You really do need to go through a fair number of practice papers using the scheme described below, in order to find the best approach for you. This means no peeking, no cheating and making yourself answer each question as if it were a real exam, including writing down your answers. This is vital since we all tend to get bored during this kind of exam practice (at least I do) and it is tempting to be half-hearted if you know it is only a practice run. Practice MCQs themselves can be found in several books covering specific parts of the exam (e.g. physiology, pharmacology, etc.) or the whole exam. There are also many unpublished collections of MCQs in circulation, some supposedly from past exams – these can be useful, but only if you also have the answers (which may be of dubious quality). The first step in devising a strategy for answering MCQs is to consider all parts of whole questions as separate questions, which can then be divided into several categories:

1 Easypeasy: you know you know the answer. You can expect to answer almost all of the questions (i.e. > 90%) in this category correctly.
2 Pretty sure: you know the subject reasonably well and although not certain, are quite confident of the correct answer, or at least have a pretty good idea. You should still get 70–90% of questions in this category correct, the large range reflecting the broad definition of this category.
3 Informed guess: you don't really know, but have enough background knowledge to judge whether a particular answer is more likely to be correct or incorrect. You should still get about 50–70% of these questions correct (i.e. more than half), although there will be lots of incorrect answers as well.
4 No idea: answering this category of questions requires a true guess each time; you, therefore, have a 50% chance of guessing it right and will average a score of 0.
5 Know too much: these questions are infuriating because although you may know the topic pretty well, you just can't tell which answer is required because of the way in which the question is structured or worded (e.g. the propofol/epilepsy question). This type of question should be in a minority since particularly ambiguous or poorly discriminatory questions should be weeded out by the continuous monitoring already mentioned.

I make no apology for repeating here my warning about the apparently simple worded question which you may misread in your haste. This error can occur for any category of question, so it is important to read each question very carefully.

The next step is to practise answering MCQ papers in strict order as above, writing your answers on a separate piece of paper. First, draw five columns down the page and label them 1–5 at the top. Next, go through the paper but for now, only answer those questions in category 1, putting your answers in column 1. I know this sounds complicated, but bear with me. Now, go through the paper again answering only those questions in category 2, putting your answers in column 2, and so on, until you have forced yourself to answer **all** of the questions in the paper. Yes, I know this means going through the papers five times, but that's the price you have to pay. The hard part is to make sure that you read each questions properly each time, although if you do this you will probably be surprised just how many misreading errors you pick up during your repeated runs through. In fact, you should now go through all the questions one final time, this time concentrating on the actual wording: i.e. have you misread any of them? Having worked through the entire paper you should now have a list of your answers identifiable as belonging to various categories of question. Now you have to mark your answers using the supplied answers in whichever book you are using, applying the traditional marking system. Mark each answer in turn, but when you finish, add up the marks separately for the different categories, giving you five separate scores at the bottom of the five columns. Now, here comes the really clever bit: look at your score for only the category 1 questions, and see how your score changes as you add the scores from successive categories of question. My guess is that your score improves as you increase the number of questions that you answer, at least up until category 3 questions. Forcing yourself to answer category 4 and 5 questions could go either way; you will need to repeat the exercise several times using different practice papers to determine which stopping point is best for you (I always ended up answering just about every question every time, except for those in category 5 which I invariably left alone). If you find that forcing yourself to answer category 4 questions consistently improves your score, it is probably because your answers are not true guesses, a concept which most of us to find hard to accept (see below). In fact, this approach may even help you by **forcing** you to decide whether a particular question belongs to category 1, 2, 3, 4 or 5, and therefore whether you should attempt an answer or not.

The above approach does take a bit of time, but is worth it since I have known scores to increase by up to a third although most increases are more modest and some people's score actually goes down using this approach. It is also possible, of course, that any improvement is simply a reflection of the amount of MCQ practice involved, rather than any specific change in technique. Also, it can be difficult overcoming your natural aversion to 'guessing' although what we tend to remember as a guess may not actually refer to the true situation. The trouble is, any question with an element of guesswork gets stored in our memory in one of two ways, depending on whether the answer turns out to be right or wrong, and this reinforces our built in conviction that guessing is bad. For example, when discovering our answer was wrong we curse and say 'I shouldn't have guessed', but if it was right, we say to ourselves 'that wasn't really a guess; I knew it all the time'. It can, therefore, be quite difficult to get used to the idea of allowing yourself to answer questions other than those in category 1 above, but again, I'd strongly recommend you give it a go.

Whichever approach you eventually go for, you should always start with the questions you have the best chance of getting right, i.e. starting with category 1 and then going through the categories in order, so that if you do run out of time, at least you have already scored the bulk of your points. I should point out here that successive statements from the College have stressed the importance of **not** guessing MCQs, based on the exam results they have obtained. I suspect that this conclusion has been reached from analysis of discriminatory questions mentioned at the beginning of this chapter, but I still maintain that it is the **definition** of what a guess entails that is the critical factor, and therefore urge you to try the above technique at least a few times before abandoning it. You yourself will only know how the technique works for you by giving it a good go and persevering with a few practice papers.

One further practical point: always allow yourself enough time (about 10–15 minutes) to transfer your answers to the computer card, since you won't score anything if you don't do this. Some advocate doing this as you go along (e.g. answering all category 1 questions and transferring them, then going through category 2, etc.); I personally would leave transferring your answers until you finished, although if you are one of those people who always run out of time in MCQ papers, perhaps you should consider transferring them as you go along. Transferring itself requires particular care and attention; allowing yourself to get out of sync can result in even a perfect score being well and truly cocked up. Make sure you check the question number on the paper with the corresponding number on the computer card at regular intervals, say every 10 questions or so. Transfer of answers is also a good time for one final check of each question and answer (still for looking for those misreadings), although it should be uncommon to change an answer at this late stage.

Revision

Once you have found your best technique for answering the questions, there are really only two ways to revise for the MCQ paper: practice MCQs from books etc. and improve your general depth of knowledge by general revision. Both of these are things which you must do. To make it less tedious, it often helps to go over MCQs with a colleague, as with other parts of the exam. As described in Chapter 2, it may also help to rotate between practising MCQ papers and covering topics, picking up where you left off last time.

4
Essays

Once the scourge of the written exam and the cause of pro-longed carpal spasm, the essay questions have been relegated to history along with Althesin and *Charlie's Angels*. However, they have risen phoenix-like in a new form, the SAQ, which receives consideration in the next chapter. The perverse fond-ness which with essays are viewed by those misty-eyed indi-viduals such as myself who sweated blood over them is an interesting phenomonen, in much the same way that people look back at their housejobs with sad nostalgia (on a 1:1 rota, no food for 3 weeks at a time, regularly beaten to a pulp by their consultant, etc.). Suffice to say that I could not bring myself to exclude essays from having their own chapter, short and pointless as it is.

5

Short answer questions (SAQs)

With the demise of the traditional essay paper, prospective candidates throughout the UK (and beyond) heaved a collective sigh of relief and countless generations of anaesthetists found yet another reason to moan 'of course you had it easy; in my day...' to their juniors. However, the essay's successor, the SAQ, is no push-over, and from the early publicity put out by the Royal College and candidates' reports, still requires fast thinking and speedy writing. In fact, some of the sample short answers published by the Royal College look remarkably similar to traditional essays, except there are now twelve of them instead of ten (and they're all compulsory whereas you had a choice of six in the old days). On the good side, they only appear in the Final exam, so at least you don't have to worry about them until later. In fact, Primary candidates can learn a lot about structuring their answers to viva questions from the SAQ approach, so it's worth your while at least to look at the SAQ format, even if you're not going to have to face the Final for a few years. Since the SAQs are something of a new venture, a certain degree of settling in will take place and the nature of the paper will continue to evolve for some time to come (each SAQ is reviewed after each exam sitting with the aim of building up a bank of 'good' SAQs), but the following suggestions should be applicable to most forms of SAQ/essay type questions.

Nature of the beast

There are twelve compulsory SAQs in the Final exam, split into two equal halves with the answers written in two books (A and B). This is to allow each candidate's answers to be marked by two examiners in easily identifiable chunks. The allotted time for the twelve questions is 3 h, i.e. 15 min per question including planning.

The SAQs themselves cover clinical topics and each paper may include some or all of the following subjects: paediatrics, neurosurgical, obstetric, cardiothoracic, emergency, pain, intensive care, clinical measurement, local anaesthesia, medicine/surgery, and dental/maxillofacial/ENT/ophthalmology. It has been stressed that the questions test understanding, judgement and communication skills, rather than just factual knowledge. Typical questions might be phrased 'Outline/list, with reasons...'; 'What are the indications for...'; 'Write a letter to a GP/patient explaining...'.Thus the wording of the questions is more specific than the old style essays, reflecting the different emphasis and shorter allotted time.

Marking

The examiners are guided as to the requirements of the SAQ answers and have a list of the points that should be covered. Each answer book is marked by a different examiner initially; different pairs of examiners have slightly different ways of arranging things but in general, only one examiner will mark clearly adequate answers whereas the second examiner will go over any question where there is uncertainty or a bad score. Where the pair of examiners cannot resolve any differences, there is always judication available from the Chairman of the SAQ examiners. This system allows the examiners to get on with it in their own base at least initially and they only need to get together (physically or electronically) to go over the awkward cases.

Each individual SAQ answer is awarded a mark of 0, 1, 1+, 2 or 2+, our old friends from before. These marks are then converted to a truly numerical value by counting the '+' as

'$\frac{1}{2}$'; thus a mark of 1+ becomes 1.5, and a mark of 2+ becomes 2.5. The values for each candidate's answers are added up and the final SAQ mark obtained using a conversion scale, e.g. a total of 18 or less is translated to a final mark of 1, and a total of 25 or more becomes a final mark of 2+. The absolute cut-off for each final mark is determined by convention but is not cast in stone. Again, judication is available throughout the whole process to ensure that everyone is happy with the final outcome and each candidate is treated fairly. This system is complicated but is used because it seems to work and is felt to be fair. It means that as long as the number of 1+s equals the number of 2s, the candidate will pass; if the number of 1+s exceeds the number of 2s, a pass is still possible if the candidate gets one 2+.

Since there is so little room for fine-tuning of the marks, as might be the case if simple percentages were awarded (e.g. as demonstrated by the difference between 68% and 61%), some basic rules can be inferred about the requirement for candidates' performance. First, just by being there and writing a brief outline of an answer, you should get yourself in the running for a 1+ without having to put down any frilly bits (unless of course you miss the point entirely, describe something completely wrongly or kill the hypothetical patient with a terrifyingly dangerous technique). This has particular importance when it comes to the technique of answering SAQs, as discussed below. On the other hand, leaving out just one question will result in an automatic fail, since you will be unable to make up the gap. Therefore, you **must** answer all the questions, and make sure you cover the whole of each topic required, however briefly.

Technique

First, as with all parts of the written exam, you must read the question and direct your answers specifically towards it. If a question says 'Outline, with reasons, your choice of anaesthetic for a patient with ...' then you should answer how **you** would do it with your reasons – whilst a brief description of alternative methods is appropriate, a long discourse on the alternatives is not really the question (assuming of course that your technique is a generally acceptable one and you're not proposing to do the case under rectal ether, for example). However, the question 'List the advantages and disadvantages of different methods of anaesthetising a patient with ...' requires exactly that. Similarly, a question 'Describe how you would set up an acute pain service' should be answered with a description of how you might go about doing this, not a lengthy account of the pharmacology of all the drugs used to manage post-operative pain, even though this might feature briefly in your answer. This latter question would incidentally be more suited to a 'word and sentence' style answer than merely a list, as would those requiring hypothetical letters to GPs about complications etc. When practising or answering these questions, the appropriateness of your answer to the wording of the question should be one of the aspects you particularly keep an eye on, and it's worth checking you haven't deviated from the point at regular intervals throughout each answer, while you're writing it.

Practising answering SAQs should be a cornerstone of your general revision programme, as described in Chapter 2, first, because it's a good way of covering the topics and second, it may take some of the pressure off when it comes to the actual SAQ paper if you're familiar with the format. Central to your answering technique is a written plan (formally called the essay plan), which serves to organise your thoughts both for general revision purposes and when constructing a coherent written answer. A plan should be written for each answer; I always drew mine up for all the questions at the start of the exam, which I still think is best if you can do it although it is somewhat scary to spend the first 15 minutes or more of the exam writing the plans before you have even started writing your answers proper. Others argue that you should do one plan at a time as you come to each question, so that you concentrate on one subject at a time, but the main advantage of doing all your plans at once is that halfway through plan number three you will probably remember something that you missed out in plan number one; if you have already written the answer to plan number one, you have to either leave out the extra bit or try to squeeze it into your answer somehow. The other advantage of the all-at-once approach is that you get a better idea of which question to answer first – it will boost your confidence to get the easiest one out of the way first and if you can scrape a few minutes off one relatively easy answer you can use the valuable extra time for the answer whose plan is the most complicated. I accept, though, that writing twelve plans one after the other may be a lot to take on at one go, so you should experiment a few times with bunches of twelve practice questions (from books, colleagues or just make them up yourself) to see how it works and how you best work with them. One approach might be to take the two halves of the SAQ paper separately, and write plans for the first six, then write the answers out properly, then do the same for the second set of six.

Because time is strictly limited, you must restrict the amount of time spent on each plan to 2–3 min: the first thing you should do before even putting pen to paper is to place your watch at the front of your desk and make a mental note of how long you have before you must accept whatever shape the plan is in and start writing out the actual answer.

So now you have a collection of plans (or just one if you prefer to tackle one at a time) to convert into concise and well ordered answers. Having noted exactly how much time you have for each answer, you must now go through your plan writing out your answer in full (remembering that the SAQ paper allows for short answers. Thus concise statements and phrases may be acceptable where perhaps they would be less so in a formal essay). The flowing style and lifting prose of the old essays have now receded from being the main requirements of this written section of the exam, and it is the organisational structure of your answer which is crucial to a good mark. Remember, the poor examiner will have a pile of papers to mark, he or she will be tired, hot (it's a strange thing, but I've noticed that the degree of heat intolerance is directly proportional to the thickness of paper in front of you) and grumpy at the previous candidate's atrocious writing and poor answer. Any extra work they have to do because of your poor presentation skill will not, therefore, help your cause. Your task is to make his or her face light up with relief when your neat, easily readable and beautifully organised answer leaps off the page and causes instant endorphin release. The general approach and layout are covered in Chapter 2, and it's absolutely vital that you practise and practise writing plans and concentrate on their structure. Remember, your revision is for improving your knowledge **and** your writing style, which leads me on to another pet subject. You **must** practise making your writing legible. As doctors, we start out with a basic disadvantage in our handwriting skills, but even the worst writing can be improved a little if you work hard at it. I cannot overemphasise the importance of this (well, I suppose I could have put that last part in bold), and examiners' reports have consistently bemoaned the dreadful writing of candidates. Add to this the wandering left-hand margin and lack of clear structure and I'm afraid you're on to a loser. I have met candidates who simply shrug their shoulders and say 'I can't help the way I write' but my response is to shrug mine and say 'I can't help you pass'. You have to make sure that your writing is legible, in a non-psychedelic colour, lined to the left-hand margin (although you may indent certain portions to emphasise structure) and make sure also that the headings and sub-headings are clearly distinguishable by underlying or indenting as in the example in Figure 5.1.

When writing your answers, you need to keep an eye on your watch at all times, making sure that (assuming 2 min for a plan) you are a quarter of the way through the answer after 2½ min, halfway through by 5 min, etc. This write-by-watch discipline is absolutely vital to avoid major over-running on one particular question thus running out of time later on so that your last question gets only three or four lines. It means that you are aware when you are losing ground and can, therefore, make it up in good time. It also means that when you finish the SAQ paper, you will probably have a headache, aching forearm and double vision, but these are inevitable however you approach it.

Figure 5.1 Beginning of an SAQ answer showing the effect of structure and layout. The same text is written in the same handwriting (a) without and (b) with due care and attention to structure and layout.

(a)

Anaesthesia in a 4-year old year child with a bleeding tonsil 10 hours after tonsillectomy
   Haemorrhage following tonsillectomy is a well known complication of the procedure and is usually caused by dislodgement of a clot over a bleeding point. The main problems are related to
   anaesthesia (i) in a child; (ii) in the presence of hypovolaemia; (iii) in the presence of a full stomach; (iv) in the presence of potential airway problems; and (v) following a recent anaesthetic.
   Apart from assessment as for any child undergoing anaesthesia (previous history, family history, drugs, allergies etc.), initial attention is directed at evidence of hypovolaemia (tachycardia, poor peripheral perfusion, sunken eyeballs, oliguria); difficulty with the airway both clinically and according to the previous records; and any predisposing cause for the haemorrhage (e.g. bleeding diathesis). Intravenous fluids should be administered and blood cross-matched if not done already. Senior help is obtained, and all theatre equipment and drugs checked as for any anaesthetic. Induction of anaesthesia is traditionally done with an inhalational induction in the left lateral position (traditionally ether but nowadays halothane in oxygen, although sevoflurane is becoming popular). Alternatively, rapid sequence induction with a small dose of an intravenous agent e.g. thiopentone and suxamethonium has also been advocated in this situation. This avoids the risk of hypotension and unprotected airway associated with inhalational induction but carries the risk of a difficult intubation and soiling of the airway if haemorrhage and/or regurgitation is severe

(b)

Anaesthesia in a 4-year old year child with a bleeding tonsil 10 hours after tonsillectomy

Introduction

Haemorrhage following tonsillectomy is a well known complication of the procedure and is usually caused by dislodgement of a clot over a bleeding point. The main problems are related to anaesthesia:

(i)   in a child;
(ii)   in the presence of hypovolaemia;
(iii) in the presence of a full stomach;
(iv)   in the presence of potential airway problems; and
(v)   following a recent anaesthetic.

Preoperative assessment and management

Apart from assessment as for any child undergoing anaesthesia (previous history, family history, drugs, allergies etc.), initial attention is directed at:

   — evidence of hypovolaemia (tachycardia, poor peripheral perfusion, sunken eyeballs, oliguria);
   — difficulty with the airway both clinically and according to the previous records; and
   — any predisposing cause for the haemorrhage (e.g. bleeding diathesis).

Intravenous fluids should be administered and blood cross-matched if not done already. Senior help is obtained, and all theatre equipment and drugs checked as for any anaesthetic.

Anaesthetic management

Induction of anaesthesia is traditionally done with an inhalational induction in the left lateral position (traditionally ether but nowadays halothane in oxygen, although sevoflurane is becoming popular). Alternatively, rapid sequence induction with a small dose of an intravenous agent e.g. thiopentone and suxamethonium has also been advocated in this situation. This avoids the risk of hypotension and unprotected airway associated with inhalational induction but carries the risk of difficult intubation and soiling of the airway if haemorrhage and/or regurgitation is severe.

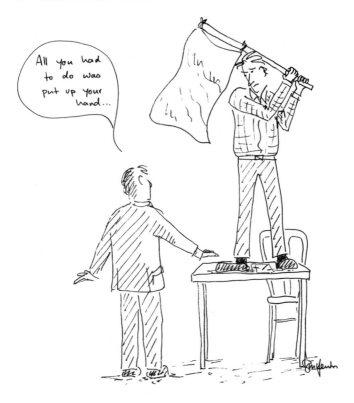

Revision

As discussed in Chapter 2, practising SAQ plans and full SAQ answers is a fundamental part of revision in general, and is something you must do. Breaking up your revision by say, doing a couple of plans one time, doing a run of six plans another time, and writing a straight set of six or twelve full SAQ answers another time, will ensure you get sufficient practice in tackling SAQs and organising your thoughts. It is equally important to practise both SAQ plans and full answers, including doing so under strict pressure of time; you need to be familiar with the write-by-clock technique when the big day comes.

6

Vivas

No doubt about it, sitting face-to-face with your examiners across a table strewn with bits of metalwork and vaguely familiar bones is one of the most, if not **the** most, stressful parts of the whole exam. For a start, it can often be somewhat intimidating to see the famous names you have read or heard about so close up. To make matters worse, you are acutely aware of your pores (and those of your fellow victims) exuding fear and tension, whilst the examiners themselves appear cool and relaxed. In fact, they may be as stressed as you are but merely better at hiding it and if you bear this in mind, it may actually calm your own nerves. Once again, examiners are normal people with normal lives and normal bodily functions, so you must try to forget the fact that they hold your future career in the palms of their hands and have the ability to screw it into a ball and toss it over their shoulder without any apparent concern, leaving you helpless and wretched with nothing to look forward to except pain and misery.

The nature of the beast

Although there are at present a number of differences in the type of subjects covered and especially in the way the vivas are conducted, the vivas for the Primary and Final exams are similar in the way they are organised.

The vivas are held over several days and there is no significance to which day is selected for any particular candidate. The Primary and Final exams have two vivas each, held on the same day, and the Primary has the added pleasure of the

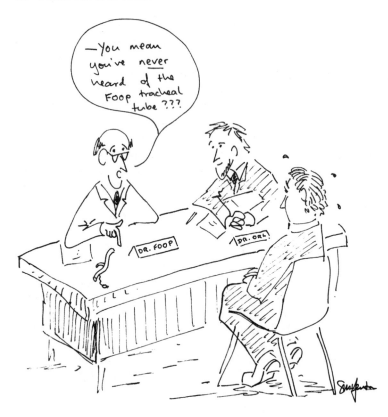

OSCE to fit in as well. Each cohort of candidates receive the same questions and great pains are taken to ensure that there is no passing on of tips to the next cohort (the subjects are changed whenever one cohort leaves the examination halls and might 'contaminate' a 'virgin' cohort). The actual subjects are altered each day; the examiners only see each day's subjects on the very morning and could be faced with subjects about which they know nothing at all. The examiners are provided with a list of questions to ask (in any order) and some structured related information to be used as guidance; the guidelines for the Primary exam are fairly loose and allow reasonable freedom for the examiners whereas those for the Final are more restrictive and rigid (e.g. including point-by-point coverage of the topics asked about). Each candidate is supposed to answer all the questions so waffling on for ages is generally a bad thing; alternatively the examiners all dread the situation where a candidate answers 'I don't know' to all the initial questions, leaving the rest of the viva with nothing to talk about. Those bright stars who are up for prizes can expect to be asked extra questions which other candidates have only encountered in their worst nightmares.

On entering the hall, the candidates are told the letter of their allotted station where there will be two examiners; each viva is split into two equal halves by a bell, with alternate examiners conducting each half.

The Primary vivas are split as follows:

1 Clinical anaesthesia (15 min).
   Equipment and safety, physics and clinical measurement (15 min).
2 Physiology and biochemistry (15 min).
   Pharmacology and statistics (15 min).

Candidates may be shown photographs, diagrams, etc. but the whole viva is essentially a series of topics/questions/ answers. The emphasis on basic safety is reinforced by inclusion of a 'critical incident' in the clinical section for each candidate to discuss and which must be passed.

 The Final vivas are split thus:

1 Clinical case: the candidates have 10 min to interpret and annotate various bits of clinical information relating to a clinical scenario, typically a short case history and results of investigations including X-ray, ECG, blood tests, etc. After a bell, they then have 20 min to discuss the case with the examiners and answer related questions.
   Clinical topics (20 min).
2 Application of basic science to anaesthesia and pain management (15 min).
   Application of basic sciences to intensive care (15 min).

Marking

Of the various sections of the exam, the orals have traditionally been the most prone to inconsistency. For example,
examiners' judgements of a candidate may be influenced by
their own values and weaknesses; one candidate's performance can affect that of the following candidate; there is a
tendency for assessors to cluster scores around the middle;
candidates' marks may be influenced by the examiners' hawkish or dovish inclinations; and examiners may be wrong about
factual matters. All these are tackled in the new, structured
and hopefully objective orals as described in this chapter and
the next one.

The same basic marking scheme as previously mentioned in
Chapter 1 (0: no show; 1: poor fail; 1+: fail; 2: pass; 2+:
outstanding) is used in the vivas. Each examiner scores the
candidate independently on the mark sheet before the two
marks are compared. Each also notes down the topics discussed whilst the other examiner is conducting the viva so
that both examiners can run through the candidate's performance together at the end of the viva. If the examiners' original marks disagree, this process may help them agree on a
final mark. Reasons for a 1 or 1+ must be recorded on the
examiners' marking sheet.

At the examiners' meeting after the vivas, any inconsistencies
are discussed (e.g. one candidate who shines through all other
parts but fails miserably in one viva), and any score of 1 is
also discussed. Last minute decisions on a particular candidate's performance may be taken although this is apparently
unusual.

Technique

There are three areas to tackle when preparing for the vivas:
basic appearance and behaviour; knowing your stuff; and
strategies for handling the actual questions.

Appearance and behaviour

Everyone says it and I will too: look tidy; avoid loud clothes and bold colours; and get that haircut that you have been planning for the last few weeks. Your aim is to impress the examiners with your tidiness, politeness and general professional bearing, not your terrible dress sense. Although much of this relates to what to do on the day itself (see Chapter 8), you may need to plan early for some aspects (get that suit cleaned, cancel your wisdom tooth extraction until after the viva date, etc.).

You also need to apply some thought to your body language. It's quite amazing when observing the exam, just how often a candidate shuffles up, slumps into the chair with a sigh and gets the whole business off to a bad start even before they've opened their mouth by adopting a negative or defensive posture. Watch how others sit and move when they answer questions in practice vivas, making mental notes about what you think is good and what is bad. Stand or sit in front of the mirror and try to look happy and confident, yet humble. Defensive postures typically involve crossed limbs; try to avoid sitting hunched over with your arm tightly crossed across your chest. Try also to avoid aggressive behaviour such as pointing at the examiners or striking the table (or examiners) to emphasise a point, and try not to let your hands form a fist. Also, don't slouch in the chair with your head propped up on your hand(s). A relaxed, non-threatening posture is sitting upright with your hands gently clasped in your lap or on the table in front of you. Keeping your palms facing upwards suggests openness and is generally a good thing if you move your hands. Watch also how you gesticulate and move when you talk – the examiners will appreciate the odd sign that you are awake and you can show them you are listening to them by nodding occasionally, but they do not want to be faced with a windmill-like display of frantic arm waving. On the other hand, try not to appear too relaxed; leaning far back with one leg casually draped over the side of the chair implies a certain over-confidence and lack of seriousness which may not go down too well. Other things to be avoided include putting your hands to your mouth or face (suggests you are not speaking the truth), moving your eyes all over the place when you talk (suggests you are shifty) and scratching various parts of your anatomy (suggests you have scabies).

When the examiners speak, you must try to look attentive (leaning forward slightly gives an air of keenness) and when you answer, try to speak slowly and clearly. Like everything else you're reading, this is easy to say but difficult to do, hence the importance of practising in front of the mirror and in front of other people. How else do you think politicians improve their image? Should you feel really self-conscious about how to sit and hold yourself, then mirroring is a useful manoeuvre which we often tend to do sub-consciously anyway; you simply adopt the same posture as the person you are facing. This instantly puts the other person at ease and reduces the threat they may perceive in you, unless of course their posture is also threatening (in which case you may end up coming to blows). Once you are aware of it, it's actually quite interesting to observe people around you and how they sit, talk, and so on. It's also (reassuringly) not that difficult to change how you yourself come across to other people just by changing simple aspects of your behaviour.

Where to look is also very important. Making eye contact is crucial to good communication, but it can be difficult to stare your examiners in the face when you feel so intimated. A good trick is to stare at a point on the examiners' foreheads when answering a question – they will not be able to tell that you are not looking directly at their eyes. A common problem is to find your eyes drawn uncontrollably and irresistably towards some blemish or strange feature on your examiner's face, for example a birth mark shaped like the cross-section of the spinal cord or a particularly precarious gob of spittle hanging on his or her lower lip. It's only too easy to find yourself completely and helplessly hypnotised by such apparitions and in these situations it may be especially useful to fix your gaze on another, more featureless, part of the face. Failing that, you can always avoid the face altogether by focusing your stare on a point just behind one of the examiner's ears (unless of course, they happen to resemble laryngeal masks stuck on the side of his or her head in which case you've got a serious problem).

A number of courses use videos to illustrate deficiencies in candidates' presentation and it's often a shock to see just how badly you present yourself when seen from someone else's perspective. I don't know of anyone who has actively videoed themselves at home having a practice viva, but you should certainly get your colleagues to comment on your performance. Spouses and partners are particularly good at this sort of constructive criticism and leap at the chance to offer corrective advice; it's often worth the week or so of not speaking to each other following one of these constructively critical sessions.

When speaking try to vary your tone occasionally so that you don't drone on in a monotone. This definitely requires practice, since it feels quite odd at first. Once again, the only way to do it is to say the same couple of sentences again and again, trying out various ways of varying your voice until it sounds OK. You do need to be alone for this; the car is a particularly good place if you drive to work since you can devote every journey to a spot of voice practice. You should also practise speaking without using those really irritating clichés such as 'you know', 'basically', 'at the end of the day', 'we was robbed, Brian', etc.

Knowing your stuff

The basic techniques are as for general revision (see Chapter 2), but it is more important than ever to speak out loud when going through the topics when you practise. In the ideal world, you want to have rehearsed every subject the examiners may ask you about, and you should bear this in mind when you practise answering questions. As stressed in Chapter 2, you actually have to **hear** your own voice to decide which approach sounds best for a particular question. For example, imagine having to answer a question on the problem of obesity for anaesthesia. You could start with the cardiovascular effects saying that the heart has to work harder, therefore requiring more oxygen, and that hypertension is also more likely, increasing the workload further. You could then go on to discuss the respiratory effects, and so on. However, if you start with the respiratory effects, the whole answer flows (I think) more fluently: '...because there is increased body mass, there is increased oxygen demand and carbon dioxide production. However, FRC is reduced and there is greater airway collapse, resulting in increasing V/Q mismatch and shunt, which causes hypoxaemia. Work of breathing is increased by the increased demand and also by the greater weight of the chest wall increasing the supply/ demand imbalance further. Thus the patient may be chronically hypoxaemic with increased pulmonary vascular resistance via hypoxic pulmonary vasoconstriction, resulting in increased workload for the right ventricle at a time of chronic hypoxaemia, which may result in right ventricular ischaemia and failure. Similarly, the left ventricle has increased workload because of the increased body mass, especially if there is associated hypertension which may lead to left ventricular ischaemia and failure because...' This particular example is one I often use to illustrate the point about practising out loud to exam candidates since it is a real-life example, from my own early exam days, that I tried several times before I felt comfortable with my answer. Of course, I was never asked about obesity but that's not the point. Also, you may find another way of answering the question that you feel suits you better but that's not the point either; what's important is that **you** practise it until it feels right.

Only by trying various approaches, first starting with one bit and then with another, can you decide which approach sounds best to you. As mentioned in Chapter 2, you must answer a question, look up the topic, decide which parts you missed out or said in the wrong order, and practice the answer again in its improved version. When you think you have the best way of answering it, go through it once more just to consolidate it in your own mind. You can easily do this alone or with a colleague, but you must do it if you want your answers to sound smooth. By going through your list of topics, you should be able to rehearse most subjects the examiners are likely to ask, although getting fellow candidates or senior colleagues in your department to ask you questions

always throws up points or new topics you have not antici-
pated and you should do this too.

Handling the questions

The first task is to try to forget your autonomic nervous
system (despite its best attempts to interfere with conscious
thought) and listen to the question. Its amazing how often
this isn't done; if the examiner asks 'Tell me how you would
anaesthetise a patient with diabetes for amputation of a leg',
don't launch straight into a discourse on invasive monitoring,
even though it may come up in the ensuing discussion and
you may know all about it. It may often be helpful to start
any answer with a brief statement setting the scene if you can,
such as 'My main concerns in this case would be the effect of
diabetes on the various body systems; the peri-operative control of the blood sugar; and the fact that this patient needs an
amputation'. This kind of preliminary statement achieves two
aims: it tells the examiners that you have this question sorted
out in your mind in case you run out of time before you get
your chance to shine or blow it later. It also helps you set the
scene for yourself, giving you a few extra seconds to get your
thoughts in order. Try doing this each time you practise questions – you may find it helpful and if not, you can always
leave it out.

The rest of your answer should be as structured as you can
make it, along the lines of beginning, middle and end as in
Chapter 2. You should practise thinking in terms of subject
headings, listing them to yourself first, then going back to go
over each point in detail. It often comes across well to do this
out loud, e.g. a general question on difficult intubation could
be answered thus: 'Difficult intubation is an uncommon but
serious problem in anaesthetic practice, the main concerns
being (i) definition, (ii) pre-operative prediction, (iii) management of the acute unexpected case, and (iv) management of
the known case'. Subsequent points of your answer can then
address these points in turn. It can be difficult to come out
with this kind of structured answer afresh, hence the importance of practising viva questions and observing other candidates' performance.

One problem of the structured answer approach is when there is more than one possible 'tree' applicable, for example answering a question about hypotension during anaesthesia. This could be answered by the 'causes' tree: 'Since mean arterial pressure = cardiac output × systemic vascular resistance, then hypotension could result from a decrease in cardiac output or in systemic vascular resistance. Since cardiac output = stroke volume × heart rate, a fall in cardiac output could in turn result from a decrease in either of these. Causes of reduced stroke volume include decreased venous return, decreased myocardial contractility, ... etc.'. However, the same question could also be answered using the 'management' tree: 'The first step would be to increase administration of i.v. fluids (or set up an infusion if not already running); increase the inspired concentration of oxygen and quickly scan the surgical field for increased bleeding or excessive force on the retractors; I would also scan the patient generally for chest expansion, colour and capillary refill and look at the monitors, especially pulse oximeter, capnograph, heart rate... etc.'. Both 'trees' would be appropriate in certain circumstances but it can be difficult sometimes to know which approach is best for any particular question and there may not always be an obvious clue in the question's wording. If you really are unsure what emphasis is required, one possible strategy is actually to ask the examiners: 'Would you like me to go through the causes first and then discuss management, or describe what I would actually do in practice?'.

By all means drop in the odd mention of a relevant paper to support a particular argument, but it's probably best not to overdo it (the examiners probably know the literature better than you do; if they don't, they won't particularly like being reminded) or to start right off with a quote – better to answer the question as asked then bring up the occasional mention later. Remember, the examiner's list of required points will not generally include specific mentions of the literature (although it's possible if there has been a specific, massively important paper).

The flow of the viva

A situation you want to avoid is having to answer questions on topics or parts of topics about which you know little. One solution to this, of course, is to know everything about everything, but unless your name is Joe 90 you will have to rely on two other strategies: luck and steering the viva. First, you must accept that your prospects are limited – if the examiner asks about difficult intubation, you are unlikely to be able to steer the conversation around to the pharmacology of anti-emetics and the examiners will get cross if you drift from the subject asked, given the list of topics and required points in front of them. However, you may have some leeway to mould the discussion towards, say, maternal mortality by dropping 'bait' at intervals, e.g. 'Difficult intubation is especially common in obstetrics as highlighted in successive Reports on Confidential Enquiries into Maternal Mortality... (leave a short pause for the examiner to ask you about maternal mortality)'. Alternatively if you don't really want to talk about maternal mortality, you could try to steer the talk towards another aspect of difficult intubation, such as prediction of difficult intubation ('Although often unexpected, difficult intubation may be possible to predict by various pre-operative tests ....') or laryngoscope blades: ('Because all anaesthetists will have to deal with the occasional difficult intubation, it is important to be familiar with difficult intubation aids and specialised laryngoscope blades ...'). This type of strategy can be surprisingly easy although the difficulty lies in not making your attempt too clumsy and obvious; remember the examiners are not stupid and have seen it all before, and if it all goes well it's not because of your amazing negotiating talents and deceptive skills, it's because the examiners are letting you get away with it. The intentions of the above samples are all too obvious but I use them to illustrate the point; so long as your answer is well-structured and within the overall subject asked about you may find that the examiners don't mind being led a little, since the viva may flow more logically and smoothly. Once again, practice is the key. The vital rule of course is that if you don't know about something, then for heaven's sake don't mention it.

One way in which you can ease your passage along a particular theme's course is to pre-empt the examiner's next question. It can be quite irritating for an examiner constantly to
have to ask for little snippets of your answer and you can
score points by saving them the bother; the examiners
appreciate a candidate who goes through the various points
on their list without needing them to prompt too often. Thus,
if you are asked 'What investigation would you request for a
patient with ischaemic heart disease undergoing surgery',
don't answer 'ECG, chest X-ray, etc.' since you must know
what the next question is going to be. Instead, say 'First, an
ECG to look for rhythm abnormalities; signs of ischaemia
such as T wave depression, T wave inversion, Q waves or
conduction defects; and large QRS complexes as evidence
of ventricular hypertrophy. I would also ask for a chest X-
ray to look for ....'. If you are really clever, you can even try
and steer this kind of guided conversation by dropping little
hints such as 'The ECG would give very useful information
about the heart's conducting system and performance, but
there are limitations to the information which can be
obtained without further tests ...'. With a bit of luck, the
examiner will take the bait and ask about what further tests
at which point you can blind him or her with your in-depth
knowledge of echocardiograms, angiography, and isotope
scanning. Remember though, this is a moderately risky strategy and you should only attempt it if you are able to answer
questions on echocardiography, angiography, isotope scanning, etc. Also, don't try and do this too often during the
viva – you'll simply come across as being cocky and will
start to irritate the examiners. One other thing: don't be put
off if the examiners suddenly change the subject when you're
in mid-flow. This can be quite offputting but it's usually a
reflection of the examiners' requirement for covering all the
topics in their list.
Something that may easily happen during a viva is that your
mind goes absolutely blank, usually just after you have been
asked a question. This is quite acceptable so long as you
explain to the examiners that your mind has gone blank
and would they mind repeating the question, whereas sitting
there with your mouth opening and closing like a goldfish

does not win you points. A similar situation is when you say the first thing that comes into your mind even though it's not quite the most appropriate for the occasion (an example uttered by a friend of mine in response to the question 'How would you induce anaesthesia in a patient with epilepsy' was 'Not ketamine'). It's probably best to follow a gaffe like this with an immediate apology and a request to start again, which will probably be granted. Another thing that's often quite difficult to do is admit 'I don't know'. If you really have no idea about the answer to a question, it's usually best to come clean and own up from the start, rather than go through the humiliating and tiresome process of having your ignorance dragged out of you like blood out of a stone. It also gives you a chance to redeem yourself on a subsequent question. Alternatively, if you think your answer is reasonable, then stick to your guns if the examiner leans on you a little – you'll impress with your conviction and standing up to pressure, so long as you are prepared to back down if the examiner really presses hard. Be aware that you may have made a really serious error or shown a red rag to his or her favourite hobby horse (or even dangerously mixed your metaphors), and ignoring the danger signs and flogging the subject to death may actually result in your own demise by a similar method. If the message you receive is 'Listen sonny, I'm right and you'd better know it' and not, as you originally thought, 'Well done for standing your ground', the best course is to nod graciously and accept defeat with a suitably servile 'Of course, yes, I see the error of my ways' sort of response. Don't overdo it though – leaping to your feet and slapping the palm of your hand to your forehead with a yell may lose you points and spill the examiners' tea, a disaster only matched by calling a female examiner 'Sir'.

The clinical case scenario

During the initial period for digestion of the clinical scenario, you should take advantage of the time away from the examiners and first jot down the various points you think are important about the case. Then, make separate lists of the points you will want to emphasise during the viva part. For

example, you can list the salient bits of the history on a separate sheet of paper and when invited, present the case using
this sheet, rather than scan your initial, all-inclusive jottings.
This makes your case presentation look and sound smoother
and avoids the examiners noting your eyes flicking all over
your notes as you search search desperately for the next part.
You can make separate lists of the examination findings,
laboratory results and results of imaging etc. as appropriate,
and go through that aide memoir when the examiners move
on to this. Finally, you should make a list of your actual
management, perhaps divided according to the patient's general condition and its immediate management, then your
anaesthetic management (assuming the scenario involves a
patient presenting for surgery); the latter can be further
divided into GA versus regional; induction, maintentance,
recovery, postoperative care, etc. When asked for your opi-
nion on anaesthetic management, you can then launch into
your list and impress the examiners with your foresight. You
should have noticed by now that the approach to the clinical
scenario viva is a combination of essay plan and viva technique, as described in Chapter 2 and above respectively.

Revision

A scheme for preparing for vivas is given in Chapter 2. You
must practice to yourself and to other people at every possible
opportunity – doing this on odd occasions during revision for
the written exams might add a little variety, but in general I'd
advise against spending too long in viva 'mode' until the
writtens are over. However, once this has happened you
must blitz viva practice. There really is very little else to
add – there's simply no other way.

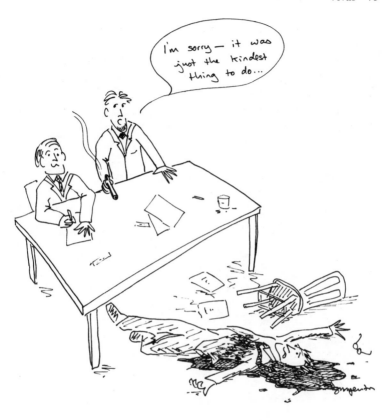

7

Objective structured clinical examinations (OSCEs)

The OSCEs are relative newcomers to the FRCA but have been around for quite a while in other exams. Although they were originally included in the Part III exam, they are now a part of the Primary only. They have the advantage of allowing fair and standardised testing of skills which cannot be adequately assessed in written or traditional oral format, resuscitation and checking the anaesthetic machine being good examples. Since the Primary is after all a test of basic anaesthetic and medical skills and knowledge, it is an obvious place for the OSCEs. Disadvantages include the large cost of organising and running an OSCE session and the enormous amount of work required in order to 'process' a relatively small number of candidates at a time. In addition, assessment of candidates' performance using a model or in the particular circumstances of the exam won't necessarily reflect their ability in other important aspects, e.g. preparation of the patient, consulting with colleagues, etc.; however it at least standardises those aspects which are looked at.

Nature of the beast

The OSCEs consist of a series of stations around which the candidates rotate, spending 1 ½ min at a preparation area (?substation) before each station proper, at which they spend a further 5 min. The preparation area is a small booth with written information about the imminent station, for example describing a scenario involving a patient or anaesthetic equipment. The stations themselves may have anatomical models, actors, photographs, bits of equipment or other props; the candidate is invited to demonstrate a procedure, check the equipment for faults (there may be some 'planted') or simply answer a series of questions. The areas tested are: resuscitation; technical skills; anatomy and regional techniques; history-taking; physical examination; communication skills; interpretation of results of investigations including ECGs and X-rays; statistics; anaesthetic, monitoring and measuring equipment; and anaesthetic hazards. Most stations are manned by one (occasionally two) examiners who, like in the vivas, have a list of required points that the candidates have to cover. Others may be unmanned, e.g. ECG or chest X-ray interpretation stations which consist of a standardised questionnaire that must be answered. There are no 'killer' stations which must be passed in order to have a chance at passing the whole exam, although some think that certain stations, e.g. resuscitation, should have a mandatory requirement for a pass. However, the possibility that a candidate might blow it through nerves and have no chance to redeem himself or herself has won sway.

The actual number of stations (sixteen in the present Primary) is a compromise between a small number allowing easier organisation and a larger number allowing better discriminatory power of this part of the exam. Having said this, it may be possible to identify certain stations as being particularly good discriminators of overall exam performance in the same way as some MCQs. The stations are drawn randomly from a bank during the week of the orals and are arranged in a similar way to the vivas, i.e. each cohort of sixteen candidates rotate through the same sixteen stations but successive cohorts get different stations. Some of the stations do not really take advantage of the OSCE format (e.g. they consist of series of questions based on some object and could thus have been included in the vivas) but are included first to add variety and second to keep the number of stations constant. There are two rest stations where the candidate is free to drink water and reflect on life.

An obvious feature of the OSCEs is the presence of actors who add more than a touch of realism to the proceedings. They are prepared beforehand with a brief set of written instructions on how to behave and what role to adopt; during the setting up and the OSCEs themselves the actors pick up little tips from the examiners and candidates about the condition they are supposed to have. The performance of the actors is generally stunning in its realism and it can feel very strange to be dealing with apparently real patients in this unreal setting – in a way they are more realistic than real patients because the latter tend to be inhibited somewhat and more friendly in exam conditions whereas the actors do the whole works: crying, begging, being aggressive, etc. I found it difficult when observing my first OSCE actor not to push the candidate aside and reassure the 'patient' that everything was alright, that her son was going to be fine; it was only the difficulty I had with my vision as the tears welled up in my eyes that prevented me making a complete fool of myself.

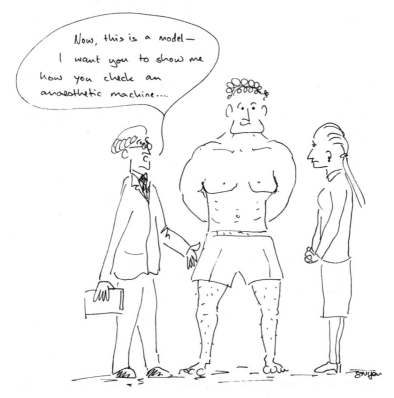

Marking

Each station is marked according to the list of required points in the examiner's checklist and is thus standardised, but there is slightly more room for manoeuvre in the examiner's interpretation of whether the required answer has been given since most stations have only one examiner present instead of the two per viva. The system is fair because the whole cohort encounters the same examiner at the same station. Each station receives a total mark out of 12–16 depending on its nature, with a minimum number required to pass the station as a whole. Some required answers or actions receive two marks if they are covered completely, with just one mark if only some aspects are covered; for example listening to the heart might require auscultation at rest and in inspiration/expiration in order to receive both marks. The ability to score marks independently for different parts of same station means that a candidate who makes a serious error at the beginning can still redeem him/herself later on. There are often instructions to the examiner at the top of the marking sheet, e.g. what to tell the candidate or what emphasis is especially required. The number of stations passed out of the sixteen stations is converted to a final score using our old friend 0 = veto; 1 = poor fail; 1+ = fail; 2 = pass; 2+ = outstanding.

Technique

The main methods of approaching the OSCEs are as for the vivas: basic appearance and behaviour, knowing your stuff, and strategies for handling the actual questions. The first two are no different from those discussed in Chapter 6; your technique during your time with the examiner(s) is also the same, i.e. answer the question asked, anticipate the flow of the session, and generally give them what they want. One difference with the OSCEs though is the extra 1½ min you spend at the preparation area before meeting the examiner; you must use this time to read the instructions carefully and anticipate the

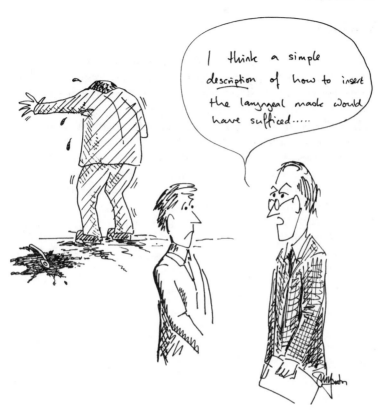

thrust of the questions, and concentrate on controlling your nerves (spend the last 30 s repeating to yourself 'keep calm, keep calm', or something similar). The other obvious difference is the emphasis on practical demonstrations and this is where you'll appreciate your hours and hours of practice during your preparation. Finally, don't forget to be polite to the 'patients': shake their hands, introduce yourself, and talk directly to them and not to the examiner unless stuck.

Revision

As with the vivas, there really is no substitute for practice. There are some subjects which are fairly obvious potential subjects for the OSCEs, such as checking the anaesthetic machine, resuscitation, invasive regional anaesthetic or vascular procedures, etc. You can cobble together your own collection or get your colleagues to set them up for you; either way you need to practice doing these things in front of other people since going through them in your mind alone will not be adequate preparation, however good you feel about them at the time. It's amazing how someone else can bring out errors and gaps in what you thought was a pretty well prepared approach.

8

Sitting the exams

Preparation

The revision and practice aspects have already been covered in previous chapters, but there are other points which are also important on the day. First, you must avoid sudden changes to your body's metabolism and intake. Resist the temptation to relieve the tension the night before the exam by going out for a curry or sinking twelve pints of Newcastle Brown; you may pay for it the next morning in the examination hall (so may the other candidates). If you're going to take beta-blockers, don't start them just before the exam; stories abound of candidates who take their first dose on exam morning, miss the bus, run to the examination hall and arrive in pulmonary oedema.

Sleep is a major problem, or can be, peri-exam. Many candidates' anxiety manifests itself as difficulty sleeping, and there are three general approaches to sleep management. First, do nothing and put up with it. This is the least risky but usually least effective strategy. Second, turn to pharmacological support (see warning above). This is somewhat risky, but might be OK if you give yourself enough time to get used to the tablets (and enough time to get off them afterwards). Finally, you can try to manipulate your sleep patterns, giving yourself the best chance of a good night on the eve of the exam by deliberately giving yourself a bad night two nights before the exam (late night movies, etc.). This can work very well and is much exploited by parents with their children, but it is a very risky approach, since a couple of mistimed phone calls or a whingey baby on the actual night before the exam can convert your peaceful slumber into a night of hell when you are least able to cope with it and have most to lose.

As far as revision is concerned, some candidates have that bandana-round-the-head, it's-not-all-over-till-it's-over approach, and carry on ploughing through their revision plan through breakfast, on the train, even on their bicycle, and stop only when they have to go into the exam itself. Others give up a day or two before ('If I don't know it by now....') and try to get by on the relaxation ticket. It seems to me that this is such a personal thing that there really is no ideal course; I always took the middle road and tried to get one last night's good revision, but also tried to flick through a few journals on the morning of the exam. It is actually quite easy to retain the odd extra fact for an hour or so, and there's the added advantage of breaking the monotony of exam preparation whilst still giving your hands something to do. If you've slipped and haven't been going through your list of useful numbers and formulae like I suggested in Chapter 2, now might be a good time to try to learn two or three items.

On the day

Despite the fact that your nerves will be jangling somewhat, it is important that you try to get in a reasonable breakfast, since you'll be burning up energy rather faster than usual. If you're one of those people who express their anxiety by re-living their breakfast backwards, then at least drink something and take a few high-energy snacks with you. Make sure you leave home in good time; you don't want to arrive hot and sweaty, flustered and certainly not late. Today is not the time to try an untested route into town or those new roller blades you were given as a birthday present. In general, it's probably best not to drive, since traffic and parking can be erratic and there's nothing worse than driving around desperately looking for a parking space knowing that you're running out of time. Try to avoid racing into the examination hall and asking to borrow money for the meter from one of the examiners. Don't forget an umbrella or sunglasses, depending on the season (or even both – this is a British exam, after all) and a collection of working pens/crayons and ruler. If you still believe in your magic gonk then by all means take it but don't forget that all your colleagues and several examiners will be watching you and you won't look like someone in control of the situation with a four-foot purple dinosaur stuffed into your suit pocket, however much you enjoy watching Barney on television.

Nobody really cares what you look like for the written exam, and there's a sort of unspoken competition amongst some candidates to see which one of them can look the most sleep-deprived, red-eyed and generally bedraggled. What you want is something comfortable; loose and light are generally good attributes whereas tight and restrictive most certainly aren't. Dress becomes particularly important for the oral exams, of course, and despite all the best intentions for allowing individual expression and discouragement of stereotypes I'm afraid you simply must toe the line and wear suitable clothes. For men, this means suits; dark colours and traditional styles create the right impression whilst loud checks, lapels wider than your shoulders and a flashing bow-tie don't. Beards and hair should be neat and tidy, clean-shaven faces should be clean-shaven and cool shades are probably out too. As far as exams go, boring is good when it comes to appearance; you want the examiners to refer to you as 'that chap who was pretty good on the physiology', not 'that chap with the Spice Girls tie who didn't have a clue', as if not knowing a particular subject is acceptable if the candidate at least looks the part but if he stands out in any way it becomes more of an insult to the institution itself. Women too have to dress the part; anonymity is the goal for you as well although in a way it's harder since you are more likely to be accused of dressing up to create an advantage over your fellow candidates. Stereotypes run deep despite our attempts to view the world as fairly as possible and I think I'd better get out of this area as quickly as possible before I get into real trouble. One last word about dress, though: oral exams are notoriously hot and sweaty affairs so you're probably better off wearing something relatively cool and risking being cold than overheating and lighting up like a boiled beetroot.

Assuming you do arrive early, you'll have time to chat with fellow candidates, get a few more calories on board, and empty any viscus you wish – although there may be long queues to do the latter. When waiting for the exam to start, keep one eye on your watch and the other one on what the other candidates are doing.

The written exam

The written exams are generally straight forward: you go in, sit down, arrange your equipment on the desk, and wait for the instruction to start. Take off your watch and place it at the front of your desk, and make sure again that you know how much time to allot to each section of the exam. The examiner will announce the rules and time limits, and tell you when to start, at which time you must turn over the question sheet and try to repress the wave of panic that usually follows when you first glimpse the topics. From then on, it's a matter of getting on with it. If you feel you simply cannot cope, stop for a minute (time yourself and count 60 s) and concentrate on your breathing, before going back in to join the fray. Whatever happens, keep to time, although you can afford to lose a few minutes here and there if you make them up somewhere else. If you find you don't have enough time to finish a whole question in the SAQ paper, resist the temptation to end mid-sentence with a squiggle going down the page as if you've died halfway through; examiners hate this and will punish you accordingly. If you do run out of time, spend the last 2–3 min getting the skeleton of an answer down, making sure you have a beginning, middle and end; for the MCQ paper, make sure you leave at least 5–10 min for transposing your answers to the optical reader card. Finally, make sure your number is correctly written on every answer sheet/book and check that your SAQs are written in the correct books.

The oral exam

In those last few moments before the exam starts, it's especially important to blow your nose, check your flies (and whatever the female equivalent is) and make sure there isn't a sprig of broccoli hanging from the corner of your mouth. Once things get going, the candidates tend to be herded around like sheep from viva to viva, which is probably a good thing since it removes one element of conscious thought and decision-making. The reason for this regimentation is that the oral exam is extremely well organised and has to run smoothly for it to work, so you should just do as you're told and concentrate on your behaviour.

Remember, there are two examiners at each viva, and one or two at each OSCE station. There may also be actors at OSCE stations, and the OSCE hall is usually full of assorted helpers and examiners wandering about making sure everything is running according to plan. You may also notice observers at any station who have come to see how things are done and should take no part in the actual exam – don't try to involve them in the discussion at all as they will be trying to avoid interfering. If you come face-to-face with an examiner or observer who knows you, he or she should get up and swap places with someone at a different station, so that everything is correct and above board.

By now, you've probably improved your body language and people skills, but it's worth repeating a few things to yourself just before you meet the examiners for the first time. Be polite and courteous; say hello at the start and thank you at the end and don't swear when you make a mistake or don't know the answer to a question. Remember that most impressions are made within the first 5 min of meeting you so make those 5 min your best performance. Resist the urge to run weeping from the room, no matter how badly you think you are doing. The examiners know how stressful the exams are and will try to help you through, but you must let them help you. Look grateful at the appropriate moments and nod wisely when acknowledging their input.

In the time between vivas/OSCEs, make sure you check your appearance again but otherwise try to relax as much as possible. If any of your colleagues invite you to join them for a big lunch and a few pints, ignore them. Keeping hydrated is one thing, but having to excuse yourself mid cross-examination to pee is to be avoided if possible (the same applies to the water that is available in the examination halls; by all means take a drink if your mouth is dry but try not to swill the whole bottle). It's also not a very good idea to try to fit in your weekly shop during the break; first, it's hard work; second, you'll inevitably be pushed for time; and third, struggling into a viva with six bulging shopping bags looks a little out of place, especially if one rips just as you sit down and spills cascades of cherry tomatoes around the examiners' feet.

One feature of the oral exams is that after a whole day's traipsing around and being grilled, you then have to sit about waiting for the exam results. Gone are the days when a man in a white coat strode into the lobby of the building at the stroke of the allotted hour holding a big book which he would open solemnly and announce in a grand voice: 'The

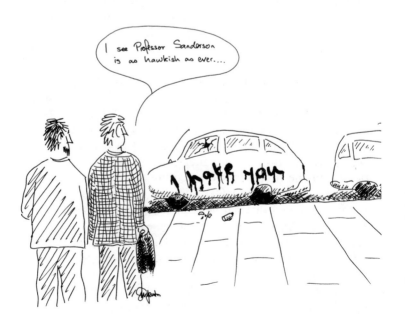

following candidates step forward and give their names'. He would then rapidly reel off a series of numbers and the rather dazed successful candidates thus identified would lurch forward unsteadily to register their names with a lady holding a smaller book, standing 30 paces behind him. They would then disappear magically into a better world of sherry and embarrassing chit-chat with the examiners (all decked out in robes) whilst the unsuccessful candidates, once they'd realised they hadn't been called (usually about 30 s after their number had been passed by) would quietly slope off into the sunset. There is the famous occasion (another urban myth or did it happen – I don't know) when the number-caller-outer gave his customary announcement, looked around and slammed the book shut before striding off stage left without calling out a single number whilst the assembled candidates stood there shell-shocked for a while before the awful truth sank in. This ritual humiliation has, I'm glad to say, been replaced by the more humane method of putting up a notice on a board with a list of the numbers of successful candidates.

Afterwards

The first thing you must do is relax, clear your mind of matters relating to the exam, and in the case of the written papers, put off your revision for a week or so. Some candidates try to jot down every question they can remember for their colleagues and themselves to go over later, either to help others in the future or to see how they did (an agonising process of rather dubious benefit). Others are either too exhausted to do this, or don't see the point. The examiners naturally enough are not too keen on this practice, but everyone knows there is a large pool of apparently authentic questions floating around various anaesthetic departments and an even larger pool in the examiners' computer. However you spend that week, though, you must get back up to speed with your revision, only this time with a different slant to your initial written-orientated revision schedule. Viva practice is the crucial element now, and you must nag every suitable member of your department to give you practice at every possible opportunity.

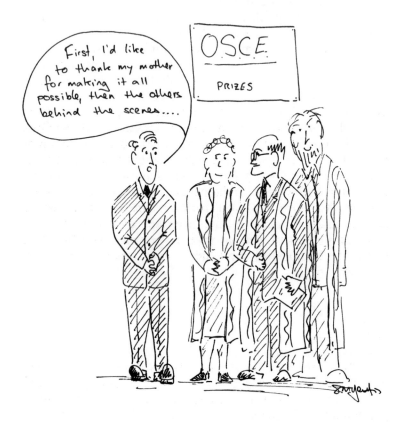

9

After it's all over

Whatever the outcome, life does not stop at the exam, although some may give the impression that it does. Once the delirium or despair wears off, it is worth giving some thought to possible areas in which to channel that energy you've been cultivating for so many months and to think about what to do next. Obviously, how you approach this will depend enormously on the actual result of the exam, and how much you're in debt to your family, friends and colleagues after those rash promises you made whilst revising (I'll do all the housework for the next year once the exams are over, etc.).

If you pass

You'll feel great, no doubt about it. And why not, you've got over a signficant hurdle in your career, especially if you've passed the Final. You get a chance to wear a funny hat and be presented to the great and the good in public, for one thing, and the calm peace of knowing that you'll never have to take another exam again (unless the rules change or you chase another qualification such as the proposed Intercollegiate Diploma in Intensive Care Medicine, an exam which had been causing great excitment with its promise of being able to call your colleagues DICs until the final format of the qualification was decided upon) is a truly wonderful feeling. A brief period of letting down your hair and enjoying life would seem entirely appropriate (some seem to define 'brief period' as the rest of their careers). Still, like an athelete who suddenly stops running, you may find it frustrating being mentally at peak fitness but with no track to run on. This is a good time to attach yourself to a suitable mentor and try to get involved in a project such as audit, research or writing case reports etc. You may find you have no interest in this kind of activity, although I'd counter that you don't really know until you try. If you **know** this isn't for you, then fair enough, but there's still your CV to think of. Alternatively, your domestic or social life may sap all your resources, thank you – and that's also fair enough.

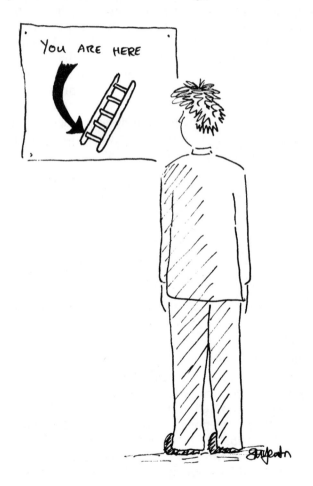

If you pass the Primary and still have the Final to look forward to, you probably won't approach your future with quite the same gay abandon, although I'd bet there's still an extra spring in your step. The obvious next move, after a celebrationary pause, is to plan your assault on the Final exam, and you need to fit it in to the exam requirements, home commitments and job movements. Current College guidelines are given in Chapter 1. Give yourself a good break but don't leave it too late, since you can never guarantee success first time and your time as a trainee is now supposed to be limited. At least you've got this book to help you prepare.

If you fail

Whoops. This can be a crushing blow, whether expected or not, and you may experience the classic feelings of shock, anger and depression before finally coming to terms with it. You do need to find out which part(s) of the exam brought you down (details of your performance in the various parts of the exam will be sent to you by post) and talk about the way you handled them, and how well you thought they went at the time, with a trusted more senior colleague. It may be possible to identify specific areas of weakness and concentrate on them next time around. Any unsuccessful candidate may write to the Examinations Director of the College for the actual marks attained in the written papers, and the comments and reasons for failure which were noted during the orals (individual examiners should never be contacted).

Two failures or a paper scoring marks of 1 in all parts results in an 'offer' of a mandatory guidance session at the College, at which the candidate's actual papers will be gone through. This session is intended to be non-intimidating although I'd have thought there's more chance of intelligent life being discovered on Uranus than this aim being achieved; however the College is serious about it and is willing for the unfortunate candidate's trusted consultants and/or College Tutor to attend (although not the candidate's mother) if requested. A confidential report from the candidate's College Tutor (with the candidate's permission) is also requested.

One practical consequence of failing the Final is how it affects your seamless training, given the way the FRCA and the training rotations are supposed to fit closely together. How big a problem this turns out to be, and how it is resolved, is yet to be seen (similar concerns have also been raised over an exit exam taken at the end of training, as now exists for our surgical colleagues. A major question is what to do with people who fail it?).

Final words

Either way, you'll have experienced something that has great significance in your anaesthetic career, and which binds anaesthetists across the country (and beyond). It's unlikely the FRCA will disappear although it will undoubtedly continue to change and adapt in the years to come. However, planning, revision and developing exam technique will always be a major part of the necessary armamentarium for surviving the FRCA.

Appendix

This is a list of topics for a revision plan for the FRCA exam. Many are noted in very general terms and could be expanded. Some are more relevent for the final part of the exam than for the first part, but are included to give, I hope, one comprehensive list. All are worth at least thinking about, although more could probably be added.

Anatomy

Aorta/vena cavae/carotids/internal jugular/subclavian veins + arteries
Antecubital fossa
Venous drainage of head/arm/leg
Spinal/sacral canal + vertebrae
Coronary/cerebral blood flow
Brain/spinal cord/cerebrospinal fluid/meninges
Mouth/nose/pharynx/larynx
Trachea/larynx/tracheobronchial tree/lungs/pleura/
mediastinum
Cranial nerves
Brachial/lumbar/sacral plexi
Intercostal spaces/ribs
Arm/hand/leg/foot nerve supply
Dermatomes/myotomes
Eye + pupillary reflex
Inguinal canal
Skull foramina
Autonomic nervous system
Diaphragm
Recurrent laryngeal nerve
View on laryngoscopy
Anaesthetic relevance of mandible/first rib

Regional anaesthesia

Epidurals: lumbar/thoracic/cervical
How to identify epidural space
Spinals
Complications of regional anaesthesia
Intravenous regional anaesthesia/sympathectomy
Brachial plexus blocks
Stellate ganglion/coeliac + lumbar plexi
Intercostal block
Paravertebral block
Femoral/obturator/lateral cutaneous/3 in 1 block
Sciatic nerve/knee/ankle block
Inguinal field block
Penile block
Median/ulnar/radial/wrist/elbow block
Dental blocks
Regional anaesthesia for awake intubation
Eye blocks
Trigeminal nerve block
Safety/monitoring
Use of adrenaline

Physiology

Function of lungs/liver/kidney
Control of BP
Effect of acute haemorrhage/i.v. infusion NaCl/moving from supine to upright position
Cardiac output/Starling curves
Cardiac cycle/ECG
Control of respiration
Mechanics of breathing
Basic cell biology
Vomiting/swallowing/gut motility
Digestion of carbohydrate/fat/protein
Hormones: pituitary/thyroid/parathyroid/adrenal/pancreatic/gut/sex/renal/other
Muscle contraction/spindles
Types of muscle
Neuromuscular junction
Classification of nerves
Action potentials
Hormones affecting the kidney
Body fluids

Immune/inflammatory responses
Temperature regulation
Effect of hypo/hyperthermia
Effect of high altitude
pH regulation
Stress response
Basal metabolic rate $+$ measurement of O_2 consumption
Coronary blood supply/demand
Cerebral/renal blood flow
Fetal circulation
One-lung anaesthesia
Control of intraocular pressure/intracranial pressure
Types of hypoxia
O_2 dissociation curve
Bohr effect/equation
Haldane effect
Alveolar air equation
Lung volumes/function tests
Starling resistor
O_2 flux/ carriage of O_2 and CO_2
Structure/function of haemoglobin
Anaemia/haemoglobinopathies
Starling forces
Coagulation $+$ abnormalities

Pharmacology

Drugs which may lower BP during GA
Side-effects of drugs
Side-effects of halothane/suxamethonium/nitrous oxide
Cholinesterases
Receptor theory
Drug interactions
Absorption/distribution/metabolism/elimination of drugs
Ionization/pKa/protein binding
Allergic reactions $+$ treatment
Thiopentone $+$ side-effects
Steroid therapy
Ideal i.v./inhalational/local anaesthetic agent (compare with current ones)
Ideal opioid/neuromuscular blocking drug (compare with current ones)
Antihypertensives
Place of N_2O
Place of halothane
O_2 therapy
Intravenous fluids $+$ administration
Antiparkinsonian drugs

Anti-ulcer/migraine/depression drugs
Drugs available in recovery/on crash trolley
Uptake of inhalational agents
Nitric oxide
Antiemetics
Anticholinesterases
Dose–response curves
Nitroprusside + side-effects
Premedication
Papavaretum
Clonidine etc.
Actions of morphine
Hofmann degradation
New anaesthetic agents
Manufacture of gases
Antiarrhythmic agents
Antianginal agents
Vasoconstrictors
Diuretics
Bronchodilators
Anticoagulants
Antidepressants
Antibiotics
Anticonvulsants
NSAIDs
Inotropes
Use of ergometrine
Clinical trials
New drugs

Physics/measurement/equipment

Measurement of volatile agents/body fluids/cardiac output/BP/blood
gases/flow/pressure/temperature/lung volumes/airway resistance/
compliance/humidity
Monitoring of neuromuscular blockade
Minimal monitoring + standards
SI units
Pulse oximetry/capnography
Scavenging
Electricity and electrical symbols/magnetism/pressure/heat
Information from arterial waveform
EEG/cerebral function monitor etc.
Depth of anaesthesia
Explosions/electrocution
Gas laws

Lasers/light
Vaporisers: classification/calibration/portable types e.g.
OMV/EMO
Ventilators: classification/ 'which do you use'/ideal type
Anaesthetic breathing systems
Tubes + scopes
Intubation aids
Defibrillators
Blood filters
Humidification
Sterilisation of equipment
Checking machines
Cylinders/gas storage/pin index/pipelines
Pollution
Low flow/CO_2 absorption
Anaesthesia at altitude/depth + equipment
'Which one monitor + why'
Oxygenators
Laryngeal mask
Draw-over apparatus + breathing systems
Pressure regulators
O_2 failure warning devices
How to prevent wrong gas delivery/excessive pressure delivery
Adiabatic/isothermic changes/Joule–Thomson effect/cryoprobe
Expiratory/one-way valves
Standard tapers
Oesophageal stethoscopes
Monitoring of cardiac function peroperatively
Poynting effect
PA catheters
Needles/i.v. cannulae
Pre-operative assessment of cardiovascular/respiratory systems
Information obtained from arterial line
Monitoring blood loss
Laplace + Lavoisier + relevance to anaesthesia
CPAP systems
Fibreoptic equipment
Definitions of mean/mode/median/standard deviation/standard error/confidence intervals/variance
How to compare two/three analgesics
How to compare exam results between medical schools
Descriptive *vs.* analytical statistics
Power/errors/sensitivity/specificity

Medicine/ICU

TPN
IPPV + modes
Weaning
Head injury/trauma/spinal cord injury
Asthma/COAD
Glasgow coma scale
Stress ulcers
Management of tracheostomy
Near-drowning/hypothermia
Sepsis
Status epilepticus
Shock + inotropes
Hyper/hypokalaemia
Diabetic coma
Decorticate/decerebrate posture
Selective decontamination of gut
Organ donation/brainstem death/persistent vegetative state
LVF/pulmonary oedema
Chest pain/dyspnoea
Arrhythmias
Chest trauma/chest drains
Pacing/cardioversion
Airway obstruction
DVT/PE
Dialysis/renal support
Pancreatitis
Severity of illness scoring
Cytokines
ARDS
Therapeutic removal/replacement of blood + products
Sedation
Cerebral protection
CPR
Transporting patients
Monitoring in ICU
Central venous/pulmonary artery catheterisation
Arterial lines/blood gas analysis
Smoke inhalation
Cardiac investigations/radiology/ultrasound
Guillain-Barré etc.
Causes of respiratory/renal failure
Thyroid crisis
Burns
Overdoses: general management/ paracetamol/aspirin/
cyanide/carbon monoxide/antidepressants

Blood gases
Living wills

Obstetrics

Physiological effects of pregnancy
Effects of drugs on the fetus
Placental transfer of drugs etc.
Pain pathways
Different methods for analgesia during labour
Neonatal CPR
Maternal CPR in pregnancy
Morbidity/mortality
PET/HELLP syndrome/amniotic fluid embolism/aspiration
Epidurals
Missed segments/dural taps/backache/effect on labour
Drugs given by midwives
Anaesthesia for LSCS/removal of placenta/forceps/cervical suture/multiple delivery
Failed intubation
Fetal distress
Collapse on labour ward
Apgar scoring system

Paediatrics

Premedication in children
Tracheo-oesophageal fistula
Diaphragmatic herniae
Gastroschisis/exomphalos
Fetal circulation
Presence of parents during induction
Interosseous infusion
Cardiac catheter studies
The premature infant
Strabismus surgery
MH susceptible child
Pyloric stenosis
PDA
Differences between adults and children
Appendicectomy
Outpatient dental
Inhaled peanut
Bleeding tonsil

Croup/epiglottitis
Radiotherapy

Pain

Measurement of pain
Pain pathways
Treatment: acute *vs.* chronic/terminal
Acute pain service/post-operative pain
Acupuncture
Opioid receptors
Pre-emptive analgesia
Post-operative analgesia after thoracotomy/ hysterectomy

Resuscitation

Basic/advanced
New *vs.* old
How to do/teach
Active compression/decompression
Defibrillation/pacing
Do-not-resuscitate policies
ICU management post-arrest
Neonates/children
Shock/trauma etc.
Airway management
Open/closed cardiac massage
New developments

Complications

Post-operative confusion/jaundice/renal failure/oliguria/
hypoxaemia/convulsions/shivering
Explosions/fires/electrocution/burns
Of spinals/epidurals
Of thyroid surgery/lasers/ENT surgery
Laryngospasm/bronchospasm
MI/myocardial ischaemia
Of individual drugs
Of carotid endarterectomy/laperoscopic cholecystectomy/hip replacement/
fractured hip
Aspiration

TURP syndrome
DVT/PE
Arterial thiopentone
Latex allergy
Malignant hyperthermia
Central anticholinergic syndrome
Nausea + vomiting
Heat loss
Barotrauma
Positioning of patient
Nerve damage during anaesthesia
Fat/air/amniotic fluid embolism
Respiratory obstruction
Of intubation/IPPV
Adverse drug reactions
Awareness
Of CVP/PA/arterial lines
Pneumothorax
Peroperative blood loss
Hypo/hypercapnia
Contamination of equipment
Peroperative arrhythmias/hypotension/hypertension/hypoxia
Needlestick injuries
Of blood transfusion
CEPOD/maternal mortality/critical incident reporting

Management of...

Dystrophia myotonica/myasthenia gravis
Marfan's
Carcinoid
Phaeochromocytoma
Acromegaly
Cushing's
Hepatic/renal failure
Transplant surgery
Sleep apnoea
Ankylosing spondylitis
Hyper/hypokalaemia/-natraemia/-calcaemia
Hypovolaemia
CABG
Major trauma
Overdose for stomach washout
Valvular heart disease
Bronchoscopy
Spinal surgery

Cardiac failure
Renal transplantation
Stridor
Laser to larynx
Hip replacement/fracture
Diabetes
Porphyria
Thyroidectomy
Problems of obesity
Rheumatoid arthritis
Aortic aneurysm
Emergency surgery
Uncontrolled hypertension
Recent MI/IHD
Angina in anaesthetic room
Outpatient dental
Bronchopleural fistula
Difficult/failed intubation
Craniotomy
Penetrating eye injury
Laryngscopy/laryngectomy
Fractured jaw
Skin graft for burns
Asthma/COAD
Sickle cell
Respiratory failure + acute abdomen
Amputation
Oesophagectomy/achalasia
Cataract extraction
Elderly/alcoholic
Carotid endarterectomy
Hypertensive patients
HIV-positive patient
ENT/dental anaesthesia
Lobectomy for carcinoma/upper fluid-filled cavity
Fixation fractured neck
TURP
Pacemakers
Laparoscopy
Chest trauma
Bowel obstruction
'Patient whose younger brother died under GA'
MAOIs/anticoagulants
Previous CABG
ECT/cardioversion
Epileptic for day-case surgery
Suxamethonium apnoea + acute abdomen
Hiatus hernia

Abdominal pain in anaesthetic room
Alcoholic/drug addict

Other

Pre-operative investigations/ASA scoring
How to design/set up ICU/recovery/day unit/epidural service/acute pain service
Indications for tracheal intubation
Sellick's manoeuvre
Assessment of recovery + reasons for delay
ATLS training
Advantages/disadvantages of day surgery
Consent
Audit/quality assurance
Research
Nil-by-mouth policies
Pre-operative assessment including airway
Major advances in the last 20 years
Smoking
Cost of anaesthesia
When to transfuse?

Index

ANAESTHESIA A-Z: AN ENCYCLOPAEDIA OF PRINCIPLES AND PRACTICE

S Yentis BSc MD BS FRCS Consulting Anaesthetist, Chelsea and Westminster Hospital, London, UK

N Hirsch MB BS FRCA Consultant Anaesthetist and Honorary Senior Lecturer, The National Hospital for Neurology and Neurosurgery, Queen Street, London, UK

G Smith BM FRCA Consultant Anaesthetist and Director of Intensive Care Services, Queen Alexandra Hospital, Portsmouth, UK

An encyclopaedic source of information on all aspects of anaesthesia and pain control in a concise, alphabetical format.

'. . . a huge amount of easily accessible and readable, factual information on all aspects of anaesthesia in a single volume.' *Anaesthesia*

'The information presented is up-to-date, practical and clinically relevant . . . anaesthetists in general and examination candidates in particular may find it valuable as a spot check for current knowledge'. *British Medical Journal*

'I can recommend this book to all libraries and to those candidates who want to be able to converse on equal terms with even the most perverse of examiners'. *British Journal of Anaesthesia*

0 7506 2285 7 480 pp 270 × 202 mm Illustrated Paperback 1995 £40.00

FRCA: PASSING THE PRIMARY EXAMINATION

H Williams MBBS Registrar in Anaesthesia, Department of Anaesthesia, North Hampshire Hospital, Basingstoke, Hants, UK

M Hasan MBChB FRCA Consultant Anaesthetist, Northwick Park Hospital, Harrow, Middlesex, UK

M Brunner MBBS FRCA Consultant Anaesthetist, Northwick Park Hospital, Harrow, Middlesex, UK

PN Robinson MBChB, FRCA Consultant Anaesthetist, Northwick Park Hospital, Harrow, Middlesex, UK

This book is a concise companion text for candidates preparing to sit the primary FRCA examination combining the syllabus of the examination with over 200 examples of examination standard MCQ's, vivas and OSCEs.

- Syllabus explained and discussed in an accessible manner
- Precise guidance on OSCEs and vivas
- Examples of MCQs with answers set at examination standard
- Complements information found in standard textbooks

0 7506 3108 2 192 pp 216 × 138 mm Illustrated Paperback 1996 £15.99

MCQS AND OSCES FOR THE PRIMARY FRCA

EI Doyle FRCA Consultant Anaesthetist, Royal Hospital for Sick Children, Edinburgh, UK

P Goggin MB BS FANZCA Consultant Anaesthetist, Royal Infirmary of Edinburgh, Edinburgh, UK

This book is a concise companion text for candidates preparing to sit the primary FRCA examination and is made up of over 300 examples of standard MCQ's and OSCEs.

- Comprehensive mix of questions reflects those of the actual MCQ paper
- Questions cover pharmacology, physiology, biochemistry, clinical anaesthesia, physics, clinical measurements and statistics
- Offers guidance in identifying gaps in the candidates knowledge on major topics
- Illustrations included in section on OSCEs

0 7506 2338 1   155 pp   216 × 138 mm   Illustrated   Paperback
1997   £15.99

LEE'S SYNOPSIS OF ANAESTHESIA
ELEVENTH EDITION

RS Atkinson OBE MA MB BChir FRCAnaes Honorary Consulting Anaesthetist, Southend Hospital, Southend, UK

GB Rushman MB BS FRCAnaes Consultant Anaesthetist, Southend Hospital, Southend, UK

NJH Davis MA DM MRCP FRCA Consultant Anaesthetist, Southampton General Hospital, Southampton, UK

An encyclopaedic reference text for the clinical anaesthetist, incorporating all that is relevant within the speciality in a structured, concise and instructive way.

'The favourite British anaesthetic text, matured rather than aged, packed with information, the only book to buy. The eleventh edition is no exception to the previous high standard, you should buy one . . .' *Today's Anaesthetist*

0 7506 1449 8 912 pp 234 × 156 mm Illustrated Hardback 1993 £42.50